AIDS
IS FOR
~~LIFE~~
DEATH

**WARNING: Casual contact
may be hazardous to your health.**

Compiled by
Dr. Jack Van Impe

Jack Van Impe Ministries
P.O. Box J, Royal Oak, Michigan 48068
In Canada: Box 1717, Postal Station A
Windsor, Ontario, N9A 6Y1

ISBN 0-934803-67-6

PREFACE

AIDS is for life, or until death. This is so because today's scientists and specialists see no cure or hope for victims of this insidious disease in the twentieth century. Because of such pessimism, fear runs rampant throughout the human race — and rightly so. Multitudinous voices either sound an alarm to warn or save millions from a devastating death, or they pacify and tranquilize the public with sugar-coated placebos containing error.

My duty as a compassionate member of Adam's race must be to raise a voice of concern for the millions who face the cruelest of deaths if they remain uninformed. Only a lascivious libertine could remain silent or pervert the facts during such a globe-encircling plague.

Recently I attempted to warn every city in America and Canada about AIDS through a nationally televised one-hour special.

Never have I encountered such unbelievable and unimaginable harassment. Gay protesters attempted in multiplied instances to either have the program canceled, or if it aired, to have the content discredited. Militants went so far as to boycott stations carrying the program and even attempted to have one station owner's license revoked in a Canadian city if the program was televised. SO MUCH FOR FREE SPEECH.

Because of gay pressure within the medical profession and the media who knowingly or unknowingly twisted, distorted, or perverted the facts I presented nationally, I felt it necessary to compile this volume. It is organized simply and systematically so that the average person might have the truth at his fingertips. The information appearing on the pages of this book are documented quotes from the world's leading scientific and medical experts (or media reporters quoting them), not statements from prejudiced talk show hosts who claim to know everything from agoraphobia to zoology.

Who is right? What is the truth? As you read the facts that took hundreds of hours to accumulate, "You shall know the truth and the truth shall make you free."

INTRODUCTION

The author of Ecclesiastes states, "Of the making of many books, there is no end." How true. Multiplied are the volumes that bear the name of Dr. Jack Van Impe. So I wondered, *Should I write another treatise on AIDS?* The answer became clear. There was a great need to research and compile documentary evidence concerning history's deadliest plague.

The project became enormous as thousands of articles were accumulated for study.

The following quotes, gleaned from the vast array of materials researched, should present the unembellished facts to all whose minds are open to truth.

The documented quotes are listed alphabetically so that the average citizen can take this volume to a talk show, a school board gathering, or any other place and have instant source materials to substantiate the point being made.

I have purposely refrained from interspersing the news releases with Bible quotations. My original treatise, which can be ordered, is a scripturally packed discourse. This volume then is strictly an AIDS guide or index to quickly thumb one's way to documented facts — from A to Z.

Thus, I let the medical professionals and media reporters speak clearly, loudly, and truthfully for themselves.

AIDS Analyzed

AIDS: A Look Into the Future

New treatments such as AZT and other drugs will continue to improve and prolong life. But if scientists find no vaccine or complete cure in the coming years, the AIDS picture is likely to look like this:

The AIDS Index

People with AIDS as of May 20, 1988: **35,769**

People who have died of AIDS as of May 20, 1988: **20,683**

Proportion of blood donors found infected with the AIDS virus: **1 to 2 per 10,000**

Proportion of military recruits infected: **1.5 per 1,000**

Gay men in San Francisco infected: **70%**

IV drug users in New York infected: **50%**

Prostitutes in Washington, D.C., infected: **47%**

AIDS patients who have died: **58%**

AIDS patients who are homosexual or bisexual men: **66%**

Male AIDS victims who are both gay and have used IV drugs: **8%**

AIDS victims who are IV drug users: **17%**

People with AIDS who are minorities: **25%**

Average life expectancy after diagnosis of a white person with AIDS: **2 years**

Average life expectancy after diagnosis of a black person with AIDS: **19 weeks**

Condom sales in 1980: **200 million**

Condom sales in 1986: **325 million**

Number of states that have barred insurance companies from using the AIDS antibody test as a criterion for health insurance: **four** states (California, Maine, Florida, Massachusetts) plus Washington, D.C.

Number of states that require reporting of the names of

USA Today (June 1, 1987).

those who test positive for AIDS antibody: **five** (Colorado, Wyoming, Arizona, South Carolina, and Minnesota)

Average cost of treating an AIDS patient from diagnosis to death: **$75,000**

AIDS care as percentage of all USA medical costs in 1986: **0.3%**

Estimated annual cost of treating patients by 1991: **$8 billion to $16 billion**

Estimated AIDS patients whose care will be paid for in whole or part with federal or state funds in 1991: **40%**

Projected 1988 federal expenditures on AIDS: **$700 million to $900 million**

USA Today, (June 1, 1987). Copyright 1987, *USA Today*. Reprinted with permission.

AIDS Caused by Virus

The letters A-I-D-S stand for Acquired Immune Deficiency Syndrome. When a person is sick with AIDS, he/she is in the final stages of a series of health problems caused by a virus (germ) that can be passed from one person to another chiefly during sexual contact or through sharing of intravenous drug needles and syringes used for "shooting" drugs. Scientists have named the AIDS virus "HIV or HTLV-III or LAV." These abbreviations stand for information denoting a virus that attacks white blood cells (T-Lymphocytes) in the human blood. Throughout this publication, we will call the virus the "AIDS virus." The AIDS virus attacks a person's immune system and damages his/her ability to ward off other germs, he/she now becomes vulnerable to becoming infected by bacteria, protozoa, fungi, and other viruses and malignancies, which may cause life-threatening illness, such as pneumonia, meningitis, and cancer.

C. Everett Koop, Surgeon General

AIDS Analyzed

No Known Cure
There is presently no cure for AIDS. There is presently no vaccine to prevent AIDS.

These are different names given to AIDS virus by the scientific community:
HIV — Human Immunodeficiency Virus
HTLV-III — Human T-Lymphotropic Virus Type III
LAV — Lymphadenopathy Associated Virus
C. Everett Koop, Surgeon General

Analysis

AIDS stands for Acquire Immune Deficiency Syndrome, which is caused by the human immunodeficiency virus or HIV. This virus weakens the body's immune system, making it incapable of fighting off disease. Technically, no one dies of AIDS — but of diseases like pneumocystis carinii pneumonia (an infection of the lungs) or Kaposi's sarcoma (a rare form of cancer). AIDS can affect anyone: Men or women. Gays or straights. Blacks, whites, Hispanics. The elderly or newborn.
Detroit News, (January 10, 1988).

Death Through Related Infections

AIDS (Acquired Immune Deficiency Syndrome) is a deadly disease that destroys the body's immune defense systems and its ability to fight off some infections and cancers, according to the West Virginia Department of Health. People with AIDS get diseases that healthy people are able to fight off easily. It is not AIDS itself that kills, but the various infections that invade the victim's body after the immune system has broken down, health officials say.

Human blood contains different types of white blood

Robertson, Kidd, *Point Pleasant Register* (September 19, 1987).

cells, the cells that play a major role in protecting the body from disease, according to the state health department. Among the many white blood cells called lymphocytes are "B" and "T" cells. Some "T" cells are called "helper cells." The helper cells help the "B" cells produce antibodies that fight disease-causing organisms. Other "T" cells are called "suppressor" cells. Suppressor cells work to stop this fight against invading germs.

Usually the helper cells are not stopped by the suppressor cells before the infection is destroyed because, in a healthy person, helper cells outnumber suppressor cells 2 to 1. But in an AIDS victim, suppressor cells outnumber helper cells, stopping them before they can begin to fight any in-coming infection. This leaves the immune system weak and ineffective in the fight against disease, according to health department officials.

Steps to educate area residents are being taken through various educational programs, including the seminar at Pleasant Valley Hospital which featured a panel of area experts...

The video, "Beyond Fear," produced by the American Red Cross, covered the AIDS subject thoroughly. The video explained that over one million persons have been infected by AIDS and over half of those persons are now dead. The disease, it said, is universally fatal.

People rarely die of AIDS though. The disease destroys the immune system, thus allowing other diseases to enter the body unhindered, and persons infected with AIDS usually die of a related infection, like pneumonia, the video states.

There is no cure for AIDS, the main problem being that the HTLV (AIDS) virus changes its protein code often, so developing a vaccine against it is difficult according to the video. To cure this infection, the cure would have to rid the

Robertson, Kidd, *Point Pleasant Register* (September 19, 1987).

body of the virus and restore the immune system strength.

Matt Robertson and Karen Kidd, Point Pleasant Register (Point Pleasant, West Virginia, September 19, 1987). Used by permission.

1,000 Times Faster Than Known Genes

Acquired Immune Deficiency Syndrome is a disease caused by what is known as a "retrovirus."

AIDS is spread primarily by sexual intercourse, through the exchange of body fluids such as semen, feces, saliva, and blood.

AIDS is a disease that attacks the body's immune system, destroying the cells that normally help fight off infections. Victims of AIDS may die either of infection or cancer caused by a weakened immune system, or they may perish due to the AIDS virus attacking brain cells, causing dementia and death.

It is the only known virus that attacks and destroys the immune system. "The AIDS virus is unique," says Dr. Anthony Fauci of the National Institute of Allergy and Infectious Disease. "It has the ability to attack very specifically and very selectively the very cells that are geared to protect you." The most important cells in the body's immune system are the T-4 helper cells which alert other cells when an infection is invading the body. After these cells fight off the infection, the T-8 suppressor cells tell the other cells that the battle is over. Most healthy individuals have twice as many T-4 cells as T-8 cells.

When the AIDS virus invades the body, it enters the T-4 cell and incorporates itself into the genetic material. When another infection enters the body, the AIDS virus reproduces itself and kills the T-4 cell in the process. According to researcher Dr. William A. Haseltine of the Dana-Farber Cancer Institute in Boston, a gene within the virus creates a

Drs. Fauci, Haseltine, *Passport Magazine.*

protein which conquers the T-4 cell and makes it produce new viruses at a rapid pace. This speeding-up process "prematurely ages the cell, and sends it to a premature death."

At present there are numerous experimental drugs under development to conquer the AIDS virus, but no cure is in sight. The virus is especially dangerous because of its ability to mutate or change form. A vaccine developed for AIDS would quickly become useless once the virus does change its form. As Dr. Haseltine has noted, "Nobody would have thought this level of transcription (gene activity) was possible before we did these studies. We were shocked. It's about 1,000 times faster than the...genes we know about. It's one of the reasons this virus can be transmitted so easily from person to person."

Dr. Anthony Fauci and Dr. William A. Haseltine, *Passport Magazine.*

So Tiny That 230 Million of the AIDS Virus Fit Into a Period Mark at the End of a Sentence.

Let's look at the AIDS virus villain. He's so tiny that he'll fit inside the period at the end of a newspaper sentence — along with 230 million others just like him. Formerly they called him "HTLV-III" (Human T-Lymphotropic Virus, Type Three). Now, by international agreement, he's been renamed "HIV" (Human Immunodeficiency Virus), which simply means he renders the immune system deficient — unable to function effectively in its customary task of defending the body against invading disease-causing microorganisms called germs.

For the infected individual, the whole process is a one-way avenue to a most uncomfortable death. As a result of the progressive destruction of the T-4 "Command center" cells, and the "palace guard" macrophage cells, and the neutralization of the B cells, the defensive arsenal of the

Dr. Rowe, AIDS Prevention Institute.

immune system is at some point rendered ineffective. HIV has a victory celebration.

New "opportunistic" infections now move in for the kill: viruses, bacteria, fungi, protozoans, parasites, malignancies. Like ravenous wild wolves attacking a wounded, defenseless deer, they lunge relentlessly, reducing the victim to a wasted shadow of his or her former self. Infants, children, beautiful women, men — all types, young and old, moral and immoral, saints and sinners — now walk that shadowy corridor of death in increasing numbers.

From all indications, the death-dealing holocaust will continue its inexorable spread throughout the nation and the world, largely unnoticed, like a mighty, silent, global explosion in slow motion. No person on the Planet Earth will evade the "fallout" in one form or another — personal, economic, social, institutional, or political.

All of which places a high responsibility on all concerned Americans. First, we must become well informed and pass along solid facts about Mr. HIV to our children, grandchildren, friends, and neighbors. Secondly, we must encourage and assist pastors, employers, educational administrators, and other leaders to assimilate vital facts about the AIDS epidemic and to make the best preventive information available to all persons residing in their local community. Finally, we must reach out in compassionate ministry to those who have entered that dark narrowing corridor.

Dr. H. Edward Rowe, President of National AIDS Prevention Institute (Washington National Headquarters, P.O. Box 2500, Culpepper, Virginia 22701).

Area Teen May Have Died From AIDS in 1969

Long before Robert R. of St. Louis finally entered the hospital, his body had begun to fail him in many ways.

For nearly two years, his lower legs and genitals had been swollen. Since then Robert, a black teen-ager, had grown thin and pale, fatigued and short of breath, and now his bloodstream swarmed with the microbe called Chlamydia.

Just when Robert's condition seemed to have stabilized, his breathing became more labored and his white blood cell count began to plummet. He developed a fever, went into a convulsion, and died.

The parade of doctors who examined the young man when alive, who poked and prodded and photographed him for their archives, agreed that Robert's immune system had somehow ceased to function.

But none of them could offer a clue as to why.

None, that is, until Dr. William Drake, the pathologist who performed the autopsy, discovered something odd: a small, purplish lesion on the boy's left thigh and several similar growths in the soft tissue inside his body.

In Drake's autopsy report, he concluded that the lesions were a malignant tumor called Kaposi's sarcoma, a rare brand of cancer once confined mostly to elderly Jewish and Italian men.

According to current diagnostic criteria, Kaposi's sarcoma in a patient younger than 60 is almost certain to signal a case of acquired immune deficiency syndrome.

But on May 16, 1969 — nobody had heard of AIDS.

The doctors who attended Robert agreed to talk about the case in exchange for an agreement to withhold the patient's last name.

Robert's case has presented a continuing puzzle, but the

Crewdson, *St. Louis Post-Dispatch* (October 25, 1987).

doctors now believe that he was infected with the same human immunodeficiency virus, or HIV, that has since been linked to AIDS.

If they are correct — and laboratory evidence obtained last week indicates strongly that they are — it means the AIDS virus has existed in this country for at least two decades, a full 10 years before the first cases of AIDS-related Kaposi's sarcoma began showing up in white, male homosexuals in New York City.

The implications of such a conclusion are profound, for the length of time that the AIDS virus has been present may not only determine how many Americans have been exposed to it but reveal much that so far is unknown about the past and future course of the disease.

But at the moment, the case of Robert R. raises more questions than it answers. They include:

— From whom did he acquire the AIDS virus, and how?

— To whom might he have passed it?

— Most important of all, when did the AIDS virus arrive in this country, and where did it come from?

Before Robert died, he was unable to contribute much to the solution of the mystery that surrounds him.

"He was the typical 15-year-old who is not going to talk to adults, especially when I'm white and he's black," said Memory Elvin-Lewis, a microbiologist at Washington University who followed Robert's decline for more than a year.

"He was not a communicative individual. He knew the minute I walked into the room that I wanted something more from him — more blood, more lymph fluid, more something."

Between extractions and injections, Robert did tell his doctors a few key facts: He had been born in St. Louis and had never traveled outside the Midwest. Nor, he said, had he

Crewdson, *St. Louis Post-Dispatch* (October 25, 1987).

ever received a blood transfusion.

He admitted having had heterosexual relations; according to his autopsy report, "The patient dated his physical disability from an instance of sexual relations with a neighborhood girl."

Robert was never asked about the possibility of homosexuality, but circumstantial evidence suggests that he may have been the recipient of anal sex, the variety of intercourse believed most likely to transmit HIV.

"We knew from the very first that he wouldn't let us do a rectal examination on him," recalled Dr. Marlys Hearst Witte, a professor of surgery at the University of Arizona who was closely involved with the case.

"We knew that he had genital edema and severe proctitis, which is an unusual problem in a 14-year-old boy — the stigmata, almost, of homosexuality. At autopsy, he had Kaposi's sarcoma of the rectum and anus, which is an unusual place for Kaposi's sarcoma to be.

"So if you're asking me, do I think the boy lived in an environment or engaged in practices that one would now associate with transmission of AIDS, I would say I think that was rather likely. He could have been a male prostitute. He certainly lived in the environment where that was possible."

However Robert acquired the virus, he must have gotten it from someone, since no viruses can exist long outside the body.

And whether he passed it on or not, the presence of HIV in this country as early as 1968 raised important questions about the current thinking on the genesis of AIDS.

Most researchers now believe that HIV assumed its present shape somewhere in Central Africa and arrived in this country during the middle 1970s. The theory is bol-

Crewdson, *St. Louis Post-Dispatch* (October 25, 1987).

stered by the discovery, two years ago, of HIV antibodies in a blood sample dating from 1959 in Kinshasa, the capital of Zaire.

Because the incidence of AIDS in Haiti is high, and because some of the first cases in this country occurred among Haitian emigres in Florida, officials have assumed that the virus probably passed through that island nation on its way from Africa to the United States.

One theory suggests that French-speaking Haitians — imported to Zaire and other French-speaking African nations as servants during the 1960s and 1970s — brought the virus back to Haiti, where it was picked up by vacationing American homosexuals in the mid-1970s.

Another theory holds that HIV first came ashore in south Florida with the successive waves of Haitian boat people who began landing there in 1978.

However it is constructed, a number of gaps remain in the Africa-Haiti theory. One is that the per-capita incidence of AIDS in other Caribbean nations — including the Bahamas, Barbados and Bermuda — is even higher than in Haiti.

Another is the question of why the virus was not also acquired by hetersexual American tourists in Haiti — or, for that matter, in Miami — because nearly equal numbers of Haitian men and women appear to be infected with HIV.

If some other explanation for the passage of HIV to the United States must be constructed on the strength of the case of Robert R., an explanation also must be found for the fact that white male homosexuals — who make up two-thirds of all AIDS victims — did not begin to sicken and die in large numbers until the late 1970s.

So perplexing was the case of Robert R. that two of the doctors who attended his autopsy took samples of his blood

Crewdson, *St. Louis Post-Dispatch* (October 25, 1987).

and tissue back to their laboratory freezers, along with the faint hope that science might someday tell them what to look for.

One was Elvin-Lewis, then a newly minted Ph.D., who had just finished a doctoral dissertation on a little-known sexually transmitted disease named, like the microbe, Chlamydia.

"He was my first patient," Elvin-Lewis recalled in a recent interview, "and I couldn't believe what I was seeing. He was a bag of producing Chlamydia. His antibodies were so low that nobody could understand it."

"The case sure was consistent with some kind of virus knockdown of the immune system," said Drake, the pathologist, who is now retired.

"The Chlamydia, for instance, shouldn't have been in his blood. Chlamydia should stick to the site where it enters the body."

Another who watched Robert's progress with great interest was Marlys Witte, then a young thoracic surgeon who — with her husband, Charles, a physician — had become intrigued by the apparent obstruction of the boy's lymphatic system.

"When he died, Marlys and I just stood there and took everything," said Elvin-Lewis. "Blood and lymph and tissue and you-name-it."

For two decades the samples were kept in cold storage, some of them in Elvin-Lewis' laboratory in St. Louis, the others by Witte at the University of Arizona.

The case remained so sufficiently perplexing that Elvin-Lewis, the Wittes, Dr. William Cole, and some of the others involved reported the enigma in a medical journal article in 1973. And there it might have ended, as the co-authors paths to teaching and research.

Crewdson, *St. Louis Post-Dispatch* (October 25, 1987).

AIDS Articles

Elvin-Lewis became chairman of the microbiology department at the Washington University Dental School. The Wittes moved to Tucson. Cole gave up his post as chief of surgery at Barnes Hospital to open a practice in Sedalia, MO., and Drake went on doing autopsies.

But the case of Robert R. stayed in the back of Marlys Witte's mind.

"I'm not someone who's devoted my whole life to AIDS," she said in an interview. "This was an incidental patient, coming in with something I deal with on a regular basis — lymphedema. But I have always thought this was an important case, and I did the best thing. I saved everything."

In 1984, as AIDS was moving to the forefront of U.S. medical research, Witte decided that some of Robert's samples should be thawed and tested.

Antibodies were found to Herpes simplex, Cytomegalovirus and Epstein-Barr disease, three viruses that — along with bacterial Chlamydia — are common among homosexual men, especially those with AIDS.

At the time, researchers lacked a way to test for antibody to HIV, which represents nearly irrefutable evidence of exposure to the virus.

"I thought that I would just sit until techniques were better, so that I would have my best shot at really documenting it," Witte said.

"We felt we had so little fluid that we were going to save what we had and do everything at once."

Early last year, after sensitive HIV antibody tests had become available, Witte called Elvin-Lewis to ask whether she had saved any of the samples she had taken from Robert.

"She turned out to be as much of a pack rat as I am," Witte said. "So I said, 'Send me everything you've got.'"

In June, Witte sent a half-teaspoon of Robert's blood and

Crewdson, *St. Louis Post-Dispatch* (October 25, 1987).

a few specks of tissue to Dr. Arthur Gottlieb, a friend and colleague who heads the microbiology department at the Tulane University Medical School.

"I thought that things were at a stage where, if there was going to be something to be found, we would be able to find it now," Witte said.

At Tulane, the samples from Robert were given over for testing to Dr. Robert Garry, an associate professor of microbiology and colleague of Gottlieb.

The test chosen by Garry to search for the presence of HIV antibody was the Western Blot, the most specific and sensitive of the antibody tests now in general use.

The Western Blot is so sensitive that the Pentagon, which is testing millions of new recruits and in-service personnel for AIDS, requires evidence of the antibody to just two of the nine main viral proteins before rendering a positive diagnosis. The Red Cross insists on three.

Robert's blood contained antibodies to every one of the nine HIV proteins used in the test.

John Crewdson, *St. Louis Post-Dispatch* (October 25, 1987). "©Copyrighted, *Chicago Tribune Company*, all rights reserved, used by permission."

The Fashion World's Nightmare

NEW YORK — AIDS is cutting a wide swath through the fashion industry and sapping its creative energy.

"So much talent is gone," says retail consultant Peter Glen. "New talent is emerging, but they're surrounded by a plague, which can only hurt the quality of their work."

The disease is a specter for all businesses, of course. But it is taking an especially great toll in the rag trade, where many homosexuals have achieved success. The tragic deaths of so many fashion-industry leaders portend permanent changes in fashion.

Hymowitz, *The Detroit News.*

AIDS Articles

"Along with the terrible loss of life, we're losing creativity, which is this industry's foundation," says Lester Gribetz, an executive vice-president of Bloomingdale's department stores, where several high-level employees have died or are dying. "You lose a brilliant display artist or designer, and his vision, talent, ability to create a style is gone forever — and can't be replaced. It's a tragedy."

Out-of-town fashion buyers find they must deal with new faces every time they come to New York to shop. Devotees of haute couture whisper furtively to one another that the AIDS plague is the reason so many collections are lackluster. And fashion executives debate how to deal with the dying while trying to find replacements for the dead.

The tragedy and its effects are going to be felt by all Americans, on Fifth Avenue and in every suburban shopping mall.

"Whatever happens in the fashion capitals of the world happens with increasing speed in every town west of the Hudson," says Geraldine Stutz, the publisher of *Panache Press* and the former head of Henri Bendel, the stylish Fifth Avenue retailer.

"If the fashions and presentations, the marketing and merchandising is suffering in New York, it suffers every place," she adds.

American fashion has lost some of its brightest stars to AIDS: designers Perry Ellis, Chester Weinberg, Willi Smith, and Tracy Mills; display artists Larry Bartscher and Robert Benzio; fashion illustrator Antonio Lopez; makeup man Way Bandy; models Michael Hanshaw, Brice Holman, and Joe MacDonald; fashion photographer William King; and fashion retail executives Pasquale Pagano, Steve Maxfield, and Carl Erickson, among scores of others.

The sick obviously aren't confined to Manhattan or Sev-

Hymowitz, *The Detroit News.*

enth Avenue. Businesses that have lost employees range from Max Department Stores in St. Louis and Dayton Hudson in Minneapolis to Parsian Clothing Stores in Birmingham, Ala., Neiman-Marcus in Dallas, and Esprit in San Francisco.

AIDS also is affecting the spirit of creativity among the healthy. "A lot of designers are either floundering or rushing to do something flamboyant and faddish, out of fear they don't have much time to live," says a New York sportswear manufacturer.

Certain fashions are being directly shaped by the disease. Katherine Hamnet, for example, is designing clothiers with special, labeled pockets for condoms in an effort to promote "safer sex" and to help stop the spread of the epidemic.

Because emaciation and the lesions of Kaposi's sarcoma are hard to conceal, AIDS "poses special terrors to fashion people, who are so focused on appearances and covering up," says William Shattls, a psychologist who had counseled apparel makers and merchants in New York.

He believes that because of all the deaths, "For many in the fashion industry, there's chronic bereavement, with no chance to get over mourning one loss before a new assault. The toll that takes on the creative process is enormous."

Los Angeles designer Harriet Selwyn was depressed for weeks — and for a time felt unable to work — after her close friend Willi Smith died in April. "He had a genius for knowing what people want to wear, and I miss his inspiration terribly," she says, citing Smith's offbeat, loose-fitting, and inexpensive sportswear.

In New York's garment district, work sometimes comes to a halt as word of yet another AIDS death spreads across Seventh Avenue. The showroom of Linda Trau, who repre-

Hymowitz, *The Detroit News.*

sents a score of young designers, has at times become an impromptu sanctuary where buyers and designers gather to grieve.

AIDS is devastating all of the arts, interior design, and architecture. But, oddly, the fashion industry has been the slowest to acknowledge the decimation of its ranks and to raise money for research and care.

"Other industries have banded together to speak out about AIDS, but so far the fashion retail world hasn't acted as a community," says Glen, the industry consultant who helped plan a big AIDS benefit that was held at Carnegie Hall. He notes, however, that the event was sponsored by window dressers and store display designers, an "obscure, minority part of this industry."

The reticence reflects a fear among retailers and manufacturers that consumers will shun stores or designers whose names are associated with AIDS. Others fear fostering the impression that, for men, fashion is a predominantly gay profession.

"This used to be a safe harbor for us — but no more," says one homosexual merchandising executive who, at a recent job interview, was asked whether he had been tested for AIDS. He says he let the prospective employer know he considered the question improper.

"I keep hearing about people with important jobs who've suddenly dropped out of sight because they're sick, but the industry is so hush-hush about it and that burns me up," says Terry McMullen, a merchandising manager at the Pierre Cardin unit of H. Cotler, Inc. "There's been no major drive for contributions or an education campaign and it's very frustrating."

Yet some executives have responded to the epidemic with compassion and caring, seeing employees with AIDS

Hymowitz, *The Detroit News.*

through long and debilitating illnesses. Arline Friedman, the vice-president for cosmetics at Bloomingdale's, vowed to stand by one of her buyers, Kenneth Probstein, when he was diagnosed as having AIDS two years ago.

"We'd worked together sometimes 12, 14 hours a day, traveled together to Europe and the Orient, spent more time together than you sometimes spend with relatives," she says. "Ken was part of our team, and that's like being part of a family."

When a few store employees and outside business contacts expressed fear of contagion, Friedman says she told them, "Don't work here, or don't visit us if you feel that way."

To protect Probstein's job and to make sure he didn't feel pressured, she encouraged other staff members to "pick up a little bit of his duties. He'd give us lists of what needed to be done, and we'd follow them. And even when we began making the decisions he used to make, we still asked him, 'This is what you wanted us to do, right?' "

Eventually, when he came to feel he could no longer handle his job, Friedman created a part-time personnel spot "that he could do one day a week or one day every three months. The important thing was to make him still feel part of the team."

As his illness worsened, "It got very hard on all of us," Friedman concedes. "We'd invite him to lunch when he wasn't in the hospital, and try to be cheerful and talk about future plans. But he could barely walk, and as soon as he was out the door, we would all sit down and cry."

Probstein died last year, and Friedman continues to feel his absence on the job. "I know how to distinguish what's great, but I can't put it together," she says. "Ken could take one rose and make it look like a million dollars. He knew

Hymowitz, *The Detroit News*.

how to create beauty at the counter.''

Bloomingdale's executives were supportive during Probstein's illness, and Friedman feels that that helped his associates get through the ordeal. More typically, the loss of key employees to AIDS has caused upheaval and uncertainty for employers.

The death last year of Ellis — who throughout his two-year illness refused to acknowledge he had AIDS — triggered management turmoil at his design company. Within months of his death, a stream of employees had quit, including both the chief executive of Perry Ellis Sportswear and one of two principal designers.

Those remaining tried to keep alive their mentor's style and point of view. "In the showroom, they'd be saying things like, 'Perry likes this color with this,' as if he hadn't died," says Judith Lebovitz, a shoe retailer in Pittsburgh who purchases Perry Ellis shoes.

Carol Hymowitz, *The Detroit News* (*The Wall Street Journal*, December 18, 1987). Used by permission.

AIDS Casts a Shadow Over the Arts

This time, the "lost generation" is literally being lost.

Instead of fleeing to Paris as in the 1920s and '30s, artists are being lost to AIDS. It has changed the creative climate of theater, dance, opera, TV, and movies, leaving them polarized between outpourings of affection and spasms of bigotry.

Rock Hudson and Liberace were just the most visible victims. *Variety* carries an average of four AIDS obituaries a week. New York City Opera general director Beverly Sills says she lost a dozen friends last year alone. And along Broadway, telephone booths are inscribed with the plaintive graffiti: "CURE AIDS."

Stearns, *USA Today* (June 3, 1987).

"It's simply part of our lives now," says New York symphonic composer Ned Rorem.

"We're not only losing our present resources, but those that the next generation will learn from," says Philip Semark, general manager of the Dallas Ballet. "We're losing wisdom, which is difficult to quantify, and we're losing art."

AIDS deaths include cabaret singer David Summers, PBS producer Peter Weinberg, stage director David Hicks, concert pianist Paul Jacobs, Chicago scenic designer David Emmons, former B-52s rock group member Ricky Wilson, American Ballet Theatre dancer Charles Ward, *Opera News* editor-in-chief Robert Jacobson and, last week, Charles Ludlam, founder of New York's avant-garde Ridiculous Theatrical Company.

So prevalent is AIDS in the performing arts that any time a major figure falls ill — or even loses weight — rumors circulate that the cause is AIDS.

Because it's often assumed anyone contracting AIDS is homosexual, many patients keep their condition secret and ask that death certificates carry euphemisms such as "pneumonia" and "heart failure."

The American Guild of Musical Artists estimates at least 50 singers and dancers among its 6,000 members have died of AIDS over the past three years. The American Federation of Television and Radio Artists says average insurance payments to members have gone up 25 percent to 28 percent annually for the past three years, partly because of the high cost of treating AIDS patients.

The disease seems unaccountably selective. The Alvin Ailey Dance Theater has lost three key administrators but no dancers. But AIDS is so common at American Ballet Theatre that dancers routinely pass around schedules coor-

Stearns, *USA Today* (June 3, 1987).

dinating home-care efforts for ill colleagues.

Last summer the Houston Grand Opera held an AIDS lecture for singers and staff after some backstage personnel died. Says company member Avajean Mears, "It's like we're in some sort of war and we hope our good friends don't get called off the front."

Sometimes fear of contacting AIDS outweighs sympathy. "Anybody who is openly gay will have a hard time getting a job in Hollywood on camera. It's simply too threatening to the sponsors of the shows," says openly gay actor Michael Kearns. "My W2 form shows that prior to the Rock Hudson disclosure, I was working a lot. (Now) I've had a hard time. I don't think that's an accident. I've seen more wedding bands on fingers, more fake wives, fake girlfriends, fake dates."

Discrimination is found in more unlikely places. At Dallas' Theater Gemini, which alternates between productions targeted at gay men and women, a show appealing to both was nixed because lesbians were afraid of catching AIDS from sitting near gay men, general manager Craig Hess says.

Thus, some artists die ashamed and alone. Opera star Marilyn Horne recently lost a piano accompanist. "He was in his apartment, being cared for by a roommate, and died without one of his friends knowing he was sick," she sadly reports.

In other cases, artists with AIDS stay on the job as long as possible. Members of the Metropolitan Opera chorus returned to the stage after being hospitalized. Pianist Jacobs made his last record while going blind and feeling so weak he could record only in 10-minute takes.

"When a family member is sick, there's a great deal of rallying, and when you're in a show together, it really is

Stearns, *USA Today* (June 3, 1987).

family," says John Glines, who produced Torch Song Trilogy on Broadway and kept actor Court Miller in the cast after repeated hospitalizations for AIDS.

PBS producer Peter Weinberg was sent home from Vienna while preparing Gala of Stars early in 1986, eight months before his death. Sills, featured on the show, found him lying in a darkened room, coughing and spitting up blood.

"I said, 'You've got to let me pack you up, you've got to let me call people, you've got to let me get you some help,' " Sills recalls. "He said, 'What'll happen to the show?' I said, 'We're almost done, you've done all the work.' So I packed his bag for him, made reservations."

Inevitably, AIDS has affected creativity. Many say they work with greater urgency.

David Patrick Stearns, *USA Today* (June 3, 1987). Copyright 1987, *USA Today*. Reprinted with permission.

In New York, the Suffering Has Many Faces — One-Third of All America's AIDS Cases Are in New York City

There are pockets of New York where the extraordinary is now commonplace, where AIDS has made disease and death the focus of daily life.

Along the tree-lined streets of Greenwich Village, where vibrant young men have already lost two friends or four or six, a passing hearse routinely signals the death of someone in his prime.

In the tenements and housing projects of Harlem or the South Bronx, where violence and drug addiction have always snatched the young, mothers now grieve for children who they say died of pneumonia or leukemia or any of the diseases that are euphemisms for acquired immune defi

Gross, *The New York Times* (March 16, 1987).

ciency syndrome.

No place outside Africa has suffered more from AIDS than New York City, home to nearly one-third of the cases in the United States. In the last six years the accelerating epidemic has struck 9,000 New Yorkers and killed 5,000 people. In the next five years, it is expected to kill 25,000 more.

On its deadly march, AIDS has become the leading cause of death among the city's young men and women and has placed a disproportionate burden on the black and Hispanic poor. Half a million New Yorkers are thought to be infected with the virus, many facing death, the rest shouldering a terrible uncertainty, their lives unalterably transformed.

These facts and numbers have recently gathered new force as the epidemic passes from one phase to another, from disbelief to inevitability.

Now city officials are bracing for an increased caseload in the very neighborhoods that are already reeling from poverty, homelessness, and ignorance.

Now volunteer groups and public health educators are seeking to reach into the shadowy corners of the city where drug abusers are the main bridge to the heterosexual population.

And now some doctors are learning to comfort dying men and women, their bodies racked, their minds ruined, while others shun hospitals that seem overrun with patients they cannot cure.

For some New Yorkers, AIDS is a dim reality that floats in and out of consciousness — there when Liberace dies or Federal health officials compare it to the black plague, gone the rest of the time.

But elsewhere AIDS is pervasive — sobering the homosexual community where it first struck half a dozen years ago, racing through the world of intravenous drug abusers

Gross, *The New York Times* (March 16, 1987).

at a new and alarming rate, infecting their sexual partners and killing their babies.

And as it kills or merely frightens, AIDS transforms the city, inexorably and painfully. It saps young talent from the professions that give New York its sparkle. It exacerbates the social and economic problems that weigh so heavily on the growing underclass. It shapes the debate about health care, sex education, and drug carefree days of the sexual revolution and casts a shadow over adolescence. And it tests the compassion and rationality of officials and ordinary citizens.

Jane Gross, Copyright ©1987, *The New York Times* (March 16, 1987). Reprinted by permission.

In the Middle of a War — 20 Percent of Gays Still Practice Risky Sex

"You watch yourself so closely," says Frank Folino, a legal secretary who has seen many of his friends in Chicago die of AIDS. "If you find a little spot that may just be a bruise, or if you get a cold, you wonder: Is this it?" For gay men, it is not just a question they ask themselves. For most of them, even that large conservative percentage that never enjoyed fast-track, promiscuous sex, it is the overriding issue of their lives. They are in the middle of a war, fighting not only the disease but also their fear of it and what they perceive as a growing homophobia in the rest of the country.

There is in fact, no parallel to the anguish now being endured by America's gay men, who live in every town and city in the U.S. and total perhaps 12 million, as many as the combined population of all eight Mountain States.

Along with pervasive fear, the AIDS crisis has caused a drastic change in the life-styles of those homosexuals who were accustomed to multiple partners. Most of them have

Clarke, *Time Magazine* (August 12, 1985).

altered their sexual habits to a degree that would have seemed inconceivable five years ago, significantly reducing the number of their sexual companions. A study at the University of California, San Francisco, showed, for example, that the average number of partners per month dropped from 5.9 in October 1982 to 2.5 during the same period in 1984. "It's just not cool to be promiscuous," says Los Angeles Art Director Jeff Kerns.

Because rapid weight loss is one of the symptoms of AIDS, some homosexuals think it is not fashionable any more to be thin. "In Los Angeles it's almost a sign of health among gays to be too fat," says Kerns, who has recently put on 10 lbs. "People now smile at me on the street."

But not all gays are smiling about their self-imposed curbs on sex. "It's like having a third party in the room, warning you not to do this or that," says one Boston man. "It makes the sex stilted and clinical." Others see some benefits. Gays who could never before commit themselves are being propelled into long-term relationships; they are being pushed into deeper emotional involvements. "I think there has been a tremendously constructive response to AIDS by the gay community," says Susan Tross, a psychologist at New York City's Memorial Sloan-Kettering Cancer Center, who has studied 233 gay men. "They are dating more. They are having monogamous relationships."

Others have made even more radical decisions. "I'd say that one-third of the men in our workshops say they've had no sex due to fear of AIDS," says Michael Wilson, president of Houston's KS-AIDS Foundation. Instead, some apparently release their sexual energies through masturbation, pornography, and sex by phone. *The Advocate* classifieds list several numbers that offer a seductive voice on the other end of the wire, payment to be made by credit card.

Clarke, *Time Magazine* (August 12, 1985).

"Horny? Call Your Adonis," says one ad. Sales of gay porn have risen, and videocassette recorders have never been so popular. "The party's over," said one New York gay as he was about to attend a memorial service for yet another casualty. "You just stop having sex. I now make love to my VCR."

Some have chosen to ignore the AIDS threat altogether, indulging still in the casual, promiscuous sex that initially followed gay liberation. A few are fatalistic. "I figure we've all been infected by now," says Corey Willis, a waiter in a San Francisco restaurant. "Either you're going to get it or you aren't. And worrying isn't going to do any good."

By one estimate, as many as 20 percent of homosexuals still practice the riskiest sexual behavior, which is the taking of multiple partners; some still patronize bathhouses for brief, anonymous encounters. "Quite honestly, I'm dismayed," says Miami's Dr. Allan J. Stein, a family physician whose patient load is 30 percent gay. "I've been trying for three years to talk to these people. I wonder: Am I doing my job right? Maybe I should have yelled." Says Jeremy Landau, project coordinator of a counseling center in San Francisco, "Let's face it. Some people just don't find safe sex exciting."

Gerald Clarke, Reported by Jon D. Hull/San Francisco and Arturo Yanez/New York, *Time Magazine* (August 12, 1985). Copyright 1985 *Time Inc.*. All rights reserved. Reprinted by permission from *Time*.

Man With Aids Sells Blood 23 Times Within Six Months

Mr. Helms has introduced a bill in the Senate encouraging widespread testing for the AIDS virus — testing that will help identify hazardous activities of AIDS carriers, such as the following:

A Los Angeles man in June was charged with

Liberty Journal (October 1987).

attempted murder after he sold his AIDS-contaminated blood.

"I know that AIDS can kill," the man was reported to have said to *USA Today*. "But I was so hard up for money I didn't give a damn."

Joseph Edward Markowski, 29, sold his blood up to 23 times in a six-month period.

And the list goes on.

Small towns, large cities and entire states have issued plans for blood testing and for laws preventing AIDS carriers like Markowski from infecting unsuspecting victims. Such policies include:

- A blood test of 100,000 New Yorkers to determine how many in the state carry the AIDS-causing HIV virus. Estimates suggest more than 500,000 are infected.
- A recommendation by the U.S. Public Health Service that routine tests should begin immediately for sex partners of AIDS victims, people with other sexually transmitted diseases, intravenous drug users, and others.
- A court order in Arizona's Pima County prohibiting a man from engaging in sexual activity with others without telling them he is an AIDS carrier.
- The first statewide law (in Illinois) requiring testing for AIDS when applying for a marriage license.
- A Nevada bill providing 20-year prison terms for prostitutes soliciting sex while knowing they carry the virus.
- A California bill making it a felony to knowingly donate AIDS infected blood.
- Mandatory AIDS testing and possible quarantining of convicted prostitutes and sex offenders in Minnesota.
- Approved laws in four states, allowing health officials

Liberty Journal (October 1987).

to quarantine AIDS victims determined to be endangering public health.

- "Care Cards" in singles clubs in some of the nation's larger cities that identify members as tested and reportedly free of the AIDS virus.

However, several of these actions are considered "homophobic" by homosexual groups who have begun a criticism campaign against persons attempting to preserve their own safety.

Washington, D.C. police were denounced in June after they wore rubber gloves while arresting demonstrators at an AIDS rally.

Police officials were convinced by local homosexual groups that the gloves were inappropriate during the arrests.

Such actions reinforce "misconceptions about how the AIDS vitus is transmitted and could be harmful to efforts to educate the public about the deadly disease," a release from D.C. Mayor Marion Barry's office said.

The response to the donning of protective gear angered Officer Gary Hankins, chairman of the labor committee for the Fraternal Order of Police.

He told the *Washington Times*, "Frankly, I'm getting tired of the gay community's political arm-twisting to conform policy to their own interests instead of the safety of the community...and my police officers."

In Illinois, the bill requiring the state Department of Public Health to trace the sex partners of persons infected with AIDS, was called "some of the most coercive and counter-productive legislation in the United States" by a group of sixty state physicians.

Beyond voluntary testing, civil liberty organizations and homosexual groups complain vigorously.

The voluntary test and continued education in safe sex

Liberty Journal (October 1987).

practices is good, they say, but required tests and informing intimate contacts of a victim's infection or tracing of those contacts is bad.

Nat Hentoff, writing in *The Village Voice* (New York's homosexual mouthpiece), probably shocked a few readers when he commented, "(If) identities (of AIDS victims) are known, the stigma can be crushing. It sure can. So can the death of someone who didn't know his or her lover had the virus. That is the very crux of the debate about testing: Is protecting privacy invariably worth the cost of another's life?

"Voluntary testing and education are essential but they are not always enough."

But only eight states now require victims of AIDS to be reported to state agencies.

"If a physician encounters a person with the virus for AIDS" in the other 42 states, says Rep. Dannemeyer, "he is not required to report that to public health authorities. And bear in mind, that is a non-curable venereal disease. But on the other hand, if a physician encounters a person with a curable venereal disease, such as syphilis or gonorrhea, the physician is required to report that to public health authorities."

The bathhouse culture of sexual promiscuity must stop and laws to ensure they stop — to ensure public health safety — must begin soon, says Mr. Dannemeyer.

It is a civil right of the healthy to be protected from the grim and deadly disease.

Liberty Journal (October 1987).

Good Samaritan Gets Caught in an AIDS-era Catch-22

Diane was walking on the North Side of Chicago, on her way home from work, when the man suddenly collapsed in front of her.

Royko, *Tribune Media Services.*

"One moment he was walking along," she says, "then he just fell over on the sidewalk. And he wasn't moving. It didn't look like he was even breathing. The first thing I thought was that he had a heart attack."

It was early evening, there were people on the street, so a crowd quickly gathered.

Somebody put a hand on the man's chest, then a finger on his wrist, and said, "I don't think there's any pulse."

Diane, who works in a law office, hasn't had any formal training in CPR (cardiopulmonary resuscitation).

"But I knew something had to be done, so I just winged it. I knelt down and gave him mouth-to-mouth, the way I've seen it done on TV."

I'm sure that many people reading this would have done the same thing for a total stranger. But I'm also sure that many more wouldn't have. A friend of mine once passed out from [the] heat on a downtown street, falling into the gutter. The closest anyone came to him was the man who leaned over, just as my friend was coming to, and said, "Hey, you're blocking my car."

But Diane put her mouth to that of a stranger and began breathing in and out, trying to bring him back to life.

"After about five minutes, he came to. But then he went under again. So I tried some more. He came to again, then he went out again. He came to three times and passed out three times before the fire department paramedics arrived."

When the paramedics took over, one of them rolled up the man's sleeves.

"Track marks," the paramedic said. That meant puncture wounds from needles. And that meant that the man was, or had been, a mainlining drug addict.

The paramedic looked at Diane's face and said, "Miss, you have blood on your lips." He looked into the man's

Royko, *Tribune Media Services.*

mouth and said, "He has bleeding gums."

At first, Diane wasn't sure what the significance of that was. She was still shaken from the experience of having brought somebody she thought was dead back to life.

"He could have AIDS," the paramedic said. "Look, he's probably an addict and around here..."

What he meant by "around here" was that it happened in the heart of the city's large gay community.

The man went to a nearby hospital. And Diane went into a state of panic.

"I called the hospital," she said. "They confirmed that he had some kind of seizure and that we had succeeded in getting his heart started."

But the hospital wouldn't tell her what she really wanted to know.

"I wanted to know about...well, you know...As far as being a good Samaritan, giving mouth-to-mouth to a guy who turns out to be a drug addict, where does that put me as far as my safety?

"They told me they couldn't give me his name, that the privacy act didn't allow that.

"I can understand his right to privacy. But on the other hand, when you need to find out if someone has hurt you, it seems to me that I have a right to know that.

"But all they would do for me is give me some advice. They said I could come in in six months to get an AIDS antibody test."

Diane then called the city health department to see if they had any suggestions as to how she could find out if the man had AIDS.

The city operator switched her to a man who asked her what happened.

She gave him a detailed account, how the man had col-

Royko, *Tribune Media Services.*

lapsed, the mouth-to-mouth resuscitation, and what the paramedics told her about the needle marks and the bleeding gums.

Then, she said, the man at the health department asked: "Did you have sex with him?"

"Did I what?"

"Did you have sex with him?"

Diane's response cannot be printed here.

"I went through the roof, then I demanded to talk to his supervisor. I told her what happened to me and how this moron wanted to know if I had sex with him.

"Do you know what she told me? She said he didn't know English too well and probably didn't understand me."

And that was about all the health department could do for her — tell her that some mope who answers the phone can't handle English.

And where does that leave Diane?

"I'm thinking about hiring a lawyer to force the hospital to release his name and records to see if he has AIDS. But that will cost me money I can't afford to spend.

"So it looks like I'll have to wait six months and take the test.

"It's kind of a Catch-22. I help someone. And now I can be in danger, but nobody will tell me if I am or I'm not.

"I'm sure it won't happen again, but if anybody ever falls over in front of me, somebody else will have to help him. I'll keep on walking."

Mike Royko, *Tribune Media Services*. Reprinted by permission.

Look for Needle Marks or See if He Is Wearing Lipstick

A couple of weeks ago, I wrote about a kind-hearted woman who gave a stranger mouth-to-mouth resuscitation

Royko, *Tribune Media Services*.

after he collapsed on a Chicago sidewalk and appeared to be dying.

When the city's paramedics arrived, they looked at the man's arms and discovered that he was a mainlining junkie. And, as it turned out, he was not only a junkie, but a gay junkie. And not only a gay junkie, but one with bleeding gums.

Naturally, the woman was alarmed at the possibility that she might have been exposed to AIDS. So she tried to persuade the hospital, where the man was treated for a seizure, to give her information, including his name.

The hospital refused, saying the law prevented it from giving out any information on the man.

So she turned to the city's Health Department for help. She told her story in detail to a department employee who listened, then asked, "Did you have sex with him?"

And that was where we left the story of Diane, the good Samaritan. Since then, there have been other developments.

"My social life has taken a nose dive," says Diane, who is divorced.

"There's been someone in my life. I showed him the article and obviously he's rather hesitant. We haven't broken up, but I haven't seen him very much in the last couple of weeks.

"My dentist read the article and now he wears a mask when he works on my teeth. Friends who used to shake my hand no longer do.

"I don't know if I can describe it, but my friends seem different now. It's a feeling I have, a gut reaction. They're concerned about my welfare, but they're also concerned about their own. With all the misinformation going around about AIDS, I'm not surprised.

"The impression I get from people is, they look at me

Royko, *Tribune Media Services.*

with amazement, and the look on their faces says, 'Why did you do such a stupid thing?' It's as if I could have somehow known that he was an addict. Or a promiscuous queen. Some of the neighbors have told me about that. (Diane lives on the North Side of Chicago, in the heart of the gay community, as it is called.)

The hospital where the man was treated still hasn't done much for Diane, although it has tried.

They've tried to get him to come in for a test. They've been in contact with his mother, and she thinks it would be a good idea. But he's refused.

"What really infuriated me is that the hospital told me that he'd like to talk to me and they asked me if they could give him my phone number.

"When they asked me that, I was furious. I told them, 'You won't tell me who he is, but you want to give him my name and phone number? Do you think I want some junkie calling me at 2 a.m. telling me he's sorry?'

"They've offered to give me free blood tests and monitor me every three months. But I'm not going to go there for the tests because they might have some vested, legal interests in the results. I'm going to get the tests, but somewhere else."

A spokesman for the hospital concedes the hospital is in kind of a bind.

"We've been trying to get him to come in to be tested, but we haven't been successful. We've also tried to get him to agree to let her have his phone number, but we haven't been able to ask him. He's hard to get in touch with, so we've had to deal with his mother."

Working on her own, however, Diane has discovered the man's name. When the paramedics treated him, they took down that information and it is a matter of public record.

But that hasn't helped Diane track him down because, as

Royko, *Tribune Media Services.*

the hospital spokesman said, the man seems to be constantly on the move.

So Diane is going to go ahead and take the series of tests. There's no great urgency. As a state health official said, "It's not like she can go in and take a shot and change anything." If she's got it, she's got it and that's that.

Incidentally, after I wrote the first column about Diane's experience, I heard from an organization that promotes educating the public on how to give cardiopulmonary resuscitation.

The organization said that I may have been irresponsible in writing the article, because I might discourage others from giving mouth-to-mouth aid to strangers.

They might have a point, so I want to make it clear that I was not trying to frighten people into ignoring someone in need of help.

But it might not be a bad idea to take a couple of seconds and check to see he has needle marks on his arms and is wearing lipstick.

Mike Royko, *Tribune Media Services*. Reprinted by permission.

Gay Couples Seeking Rights and Privileges of Straight Marriages

WASHINGTON, D.C. — Across the country, a growing number of gay men and lesbians are not only choosing long-term relationships but seeking access to some of the rights and privileges readily available to heterosexual couples.

At least one in four gay men or lesbians — or five million Americans — now live in same-sex relationships of more than a year standing, said California author and sex therapist Dr. Betty Berzan. But no where are these relationships recognized as legal marriages.

This October in the nation's capital, several thousand

Dallas Times Herald (December 13, 1987).

same-sex couples and their supporters gathered in front of the Internal Revenue Service headquarters to take part in a non-denominational marriage celebration and to demand an end to what they consider discrimination against their relationships.

What gay and lesbian couples want, said Rosemary Dempsey, a lawyer and head of the National Organization of Women's lesbian rights program, are "Our constitutional rights to life, liberty, and the pursuit of happiness."

The AIDS crisis has shone a searing spotlight on the kinds of problems that can beset same-sex couples who lack the protection of a marriage license.

Horror stories abound from coast to coast. Lovers of men who have died of AIDS, like Boston poet and professor Ron Shreiber, have been excluded from their deceased partner's obituaries in mainstream newspapers. Others have been refused the right to make funeral or burial arrangements, to visit a lover in the hospital, or to be included in medical decisions. In New York, partners of men who have died of AIDS have been evicted from rent-stabilized apartments, because the name of the lease was that of a deceased lover, and the landlord refused to extend it to the surviving partner.

In a case that has generated considerable publicity, 35-year-old actor and costume designer Everett Quinton is suing to remain in the Greenwich Village apartment he shared for 11 years with playwright and former artistic director of the Ridiculous Theater Company, Charles Ludlam, who died of AIDS this year.

Quinton, who said he and Ludlam lived together for 12 years, essentially as a married couple, was served an eviction notice last summer.

Dallas Times Herald (Pacific News Service, December 13, 1987). Used by permission.

AIDS Articles

Homosexual's Lover Awarded Custody of His Son

The saga of Brian Batey, the boy at the center of a bitter custody dispute between his fundamentalist mother and his homosexual father, apparently ended Thursday when a judge awarded custody of the teenager to the male companion of his late father.

Los Angeles Times (November 6, 1987).

On November 5, San Diego Judge Judith McConnell awarded the custody of Batey's 16-year-old son, Brian, to the homosexual lover of her divorced husband, who died from AIDS earlier this year.

Thus ended five years of agony and outrage for Betty Lou Batey as she battled unsuccessfully to regain custody of her son.

It began in 1982, when California Judge Sheridan Reed took custody of Brian away from Mrs. Batey and awarded it to her former husband Frank Batey, because she had curtailed his visitation rights.

What the court failed to note was that she had done so for a very good reason: Her son Brian (then age 9) didn't want to be exposed anymore to his father's disturbing sexual proclivities. One time he walked in and found his father in bed with three other men; another time he found his father and a partner on top of each other. Nor was sex the only issue involved. During custody hearings, Brian testified that his father grew and smoked marijuana.

Orange County Register (November 20, 1987).

The Injustice of the Judicial System: The Pro-homosexual and Anti-Christian Bias of Some Judges

The United States Constitution is supposed to guarantee equal treatment under the law to all our citizens. Try telling that to Mrs. Betty Lou Batey, who just lost her five-year court battle for the parental rights of her son, Brian, all because of a pro-homosexual judge, whose anti-Christian bias was clear during the entire proceedings.

Judge Judith McConnell was anything but fair and objective in the hearing of this case. Brian and his mother came into her court because Betty and Frank Batey had a conflict over visiting privileges resulting from their divorce due to Frank's homosexuality. It seems that Brian found his father's homosexual activities in the home distasteful. He testified in court that he had walked in more than once and found his father engaged in such activity. He also said he witnessed that his father grew and smoked marijuana.

In spite of these facts, the judge gave custody of Brian to his father, who was living with a homosexual "lover." This caused Betty to take her son to another state where they lived for two years. Finally, with the police close behind her, she gave herself up, hoping for some kind of justice in the courts.

After some time, Frank died of AIDS and the judge assigned custody of Brian to the "lover" of his dead father, over Betty's protest. The judge made this decision in spite of the fact that this now 16-year-old had admitted in court that he was on drugs, had used alcohol, had neglected his studies, was failing in school, and was living a very permissive lifestyle in the home of his dead father's "homosexual partner." You may ask, "How could the judge make such a decision" — easy, she was raised by a homosexual father

Tim LaHaye Report (January 1988).

herself.

Betty's attorneys demanded that in fairness Judge McConnell should step down, but she refused. You might wonder how she ever got to be a judge in the first place. Very simple — she was appointed by former Governor Jerry "Moonbeam" Brown, of whom it was widely rumored that he was "gay."

Now do you see why it is imperative that we elect the right president for our country and the right governors for our states? These two officials are responsible for most of our judges, and be sure of this, a judge is no more unbiased or objective than you or I. He will make decisions on the basis of his philosophy of life. It happens in our courts every day.

If we are to have more pro-moral, pro-family judges with a healthy respect for Christianity, we will have to elect more conservative governors and a president who will appoint judges like themselves.

Tim LaHaye Report (January 1988).

The Strange Battle Against AIDS — Legalize Anal Intercourse for 14 Year Olds in Canada

One-third of AIDS cases are in Toronto, the centre of the homosexual community in English Canada. In May 1987 a Toronto woman was diagnosed as having AIDS through a blood transfusion. According to Anne Moon, of the city's department of public health, she was the first person in Toronto to get the fatal disease through means other than sexual relations with homosexuals or so-called "bisexuals." The latter are men who do unnatural acts with other men and then have relations with their wives, with prostitutes, or other women. It is this group of fornicators who transmit the fatal disease into the mainstream of society.

Campaign Life News (August 1987).

While there is a constant demand for taxpayer's money to fight AIDS, several strange features continue to characterize this so-called battle against AIDS.

First, the homosexual subculture which now threatens the welfare of all society, is allowed to flourish without restrictions. In Toronto, Vancouver, Montreal, and other cities, homosexual movies and plays continue to be hailed and promoted by the media. Some of the reviewers are themselves homosexuals, such as movie reviewer Jay Scott of the *Globe and Mail.*

No attempt is made to close the gathering places of homosexuals, their bars, bathhouses, and hotels. Prostitution, madams, and whore houses, through whose "services" AIDS spreads into the wider community, continue to bask in a glow of general media approval as legitimate or entertaining enterprises, supposedly harassed only by a small group of narrow-minded Victorian prudes who won't allow the citizens their bit of fun and pleasure.

On the political scene spokesmen for the permissive society continue their outrageous behaviour. The homosexuals' chief champion, MP Svend Robinson (Vancouver-Burnaby), Justice Critic for the NDP, attacked the government in the House of Commons on November 4, 1986, for "discrimination" against homosexuals. He demanded the lowering of the age of consent and the legalization of anal intercourse with children from the age of 14 and on. He actually moved such an amendment to Bill C-15 in the Justice Committee hearings of the House.

At the same time, the National Action Committee for women (NAC), the government-subsidized feminists' organization, presently under the leadership of Louise Dulude (whose live-in companion is social issues columnist Leonard Shifrin), demands the "decriminalization" of

Campaign Life News (August 1987).

prostitution and the recognition of its practitioners as a legitimate profession. In 1985 NAC accepted CORP (Canadian Organization for the Rights of Prostitutes) as a new corporate member.

Judges in Vancouver and Toronto, continue to declare homosexual "literature" not obscene. On March 21, 1987, Toronto Judge Bruce Hawkins, in declaring the book *The Joy of Gay Sex* not obscene, stated:

"To write about homosexual practices without dealing with anal intercourse would be equivalent to writing a history of music and omitting Mozart."

One notes that delicacy and nobility of the comparison!

Finally, those provinces or school districts which intend to fight immoral sexual activity most radically through the promotion of chastity and abstention from sex before marriage are ridiculed as promoting "Victorian morals."

In Ontario, the *Toronto Star* of May 15 reported Joan Wright, counselor at Toronto's Bay Centre for Birth Control, saying that a teen's sex drive is very strong and emphasizing chastity and marriage detracts from "the more realistic focus on using condoms." Dallas Petroff, executive director of Toronto's Planned Parenthood, attacked abstinence from sex before marriage as another sensational "scare tactic" by adults trying to control their lives. Petroff seems unaware that the tradition is 10,000 years old and was the accepted standard for moral behaviour until the permissiveness of the nineteen-sixties.

Phil Shaw, a spokesman for the AIDS Committee of Toronto, thought Ontario's proposed AIDS curriculum was confusing a health issue with a "moral message about concepts like marriage." Dr. David Walters, head of the AIDS awareness and education program for the Canadian Public Health Association, thinks students should be left to

Campaign Life News (August 1987).

"establish their own values."

While the views of these spokesmen for the contraceptive mentality and moral permissiveness are not surprising, they are revealing, nevertheless. Students are apparently better off with condoms, thus playing Russian roulette with a deadly disease, than with complete freedom and peace of mind through abstinence.

What is most distressing is that it is these groups which rake in taxpayer's money via government grants under the guise of "battling" AIDS. By refusing to accept the one foolproof method, they are actually promoting the spread of AIDS.

Campaign Life News (August 1987).

4,000 Homosexual Ministers in Church of England

The Church of England yesterday rejected a proposal to ban homosexuals from the priesthood as controversy over the issue continued to embarrass church leaders.

Archbishop of Canterbury Robert Runcie admitted that the dispute has given the impression that "the church is soft on morality."

Outside Church House, where the Anglican Synod, or congress, was held, homosexuals and lesbians demonstrated for "gay rights" in the pulpit. Some church members countered that the Bible condemns homosexuality.

Some homosexual church members claimed that more than a third of the 12,000 clergymen share their sexual orientation.

The synod voted 408-8 with 13 abstentions to approve a motion condemning fornication and adultery as sins and saying sexual intercourse "properly belongs in marriage."

Morrison, *The Summit Journal* (November 12, 1987).

"Homosexual acts fall short of this ideal," the motion said. It adds that homosexuality should be "met with a call to repentance and compassion."

The Rev. Tony Higton had proposed a motion that effectively would have outlawed homosexual men from the priesthood.

The synod met under a cloud of controversy. On Sunday, *The People*, a popular tabloid, named several Anglican clergymen it said are homosexual.

The article quoted the churchmen as describing trips to gay bars, nights with motorcycle clubs, indulgence in sadomasochism, and group sex.

The People identified the Rev. Alan Sanders as the clergyman who helped the paper "expose" homosexuality in the Church of England.

The London tabloid press yesterday was full of cartoons ridiculing the church and its clergymen.

The Star showed priests in robes putting on a fashion show. *The Daily Mirror* showed a clergyman in fishnet stockings and a wig trying to seduce another clergyman at a cocktail party.

James Morrison, *The Summit Journal* (*The Washington Times*, November 12, 1987). Used by permission.

100 Clergymen in England Will Die of AIDS Within Five Years

More than 100 Church of England clergymen, possibly including a bishop, will die of AIDS within five years, an expert on the care of the dying claimed yesterday.

But the church is covering up the extent of this nightmare because it fears offending the gay community, according to Dr. Patrick Dixon of University College Hospital, London, whose new book on the disease, *The Truth About AIDS*, is

The Summit Journal (November 4, 1987).

launched tomorrow.

He said that while accurate figures on English clergy suffering from AIDS were not available, the London-based Lesbian and Gay Christian Movement has said there could be as many as 6,000 homosexual clergy in the UK.

While stressing that the church's proper response to AIDS sufferers should be compassion, he argued that it should set standards for its own clergy if its call on society to return to biblical standards of morality were to be heeded.

He called upon the church to help explode some of the myths that surround the disease and to support efforts to establish Christian hospices to care for the dying. He said he planned to disclose some new and alarming facts about AIDS at tomorrow's London launch.

The Summit Journal (*Business Day*, November 4, 1987).

Dallas Has Highest AIDS Increase Rate in the Nation

The Dallas area had a larger percentage increase in AIDS cases in 1986 than any other metropolitan area in the nation, according to statistics released recently by the federal Centers for Disease Control in Atlanta.

(This city banned my telecast. Interesting? — JVI)

Beill Deener, *The Dallas Morning News* (August 26, 1987).

AIDS Becoming Major Issue for Indian Tribes — Navajos Tribal Legend on AIDS

AIDS is spreading rapidly through America's Indian tribes and could wipe out some of the smaller reservations, partly because the culture tolerates bisexual relationships, the chief physician for the nation's biggest tribe said...

"We are finally convincing people that the issue must be faced," Dr. Ben Muneta, chief medical officer for the

U.P.I. (Spokane, Washington).

Navajo Department of Health, said. "But you can't tell people not to have sex."

Ironically, the traditional Navajo medicine men, say it is not a new threat but one with a history in ancient tribal legends.

"Medicine men are coming unsolicited in to see me," Muneta said, adding that tribal legends tell of a disease that decimated the Navajos just after the tribe's version of the creation.

"In the legend, the disease is almost exactly like AIDS," Muneta said.

The medicine men say the only defense against the ancient disease was to live a "life of moderation." Their predecessors prescribed herbs to lessen the symptoms of the disease, but the stricken still died.

"Considering safe sex practices — it's sort of what we are saying today," Muneta said.

Muneta said the old religious ways of the tribe may gain new vigor in the next decade because the rituals and treatments may give the AIDS-stricken Navajos comfort and even reduce the stress that some researchers believe activates the latent virus.

Muneta spoke at a meeting of Indian health professionals.

U.P.I. (Spokane, Washington).

Personal Attacks by the Media for Quoting Their Articles Is Sheer Hypocrisy

(The following was a letter sent to all of my sponsors — JVI.)

The battle rages.

Two months ago I wrote stating, "At 5:00 a.m. I was awakened and God brought a word of warning to my heart concerning our nationwide TV special, 'The AIDS Cover-Up.' "

The promise God gave me two months ago as He burned the warning repeatedly into my heart is for the present moment.

First, I will analyze what they said concerning my nationwide TV special, and then I will list the media's quotes upon which my information is based. Undoubtedly, apologies should be forthcoming in light of the evidence you are about to read, but I will not hold my breath.

In Madison, Wisconsin, the station manager said, "We felt that the program was inaccurate and inflammatory."

In Dallas, Texas, the manager was honest with us. He said, "We do not want to air the program because we are afraid that Gay Activists will march on our station and require equal time."

In Harrisonburg, Virginia, the station manager said, "The program is not targeted for the people who are watching this station."

In Charlotte, North Carolina, the story is shocking to say the least. The station pulled the plug before they ever got to the message on AIDS. After having received over 500 calls from angry citizens protesting the cancellation of the program, the station manager made public apology to Jack Van

JVI Progress Report (October 1987).

Alarming AIDS Announcements

Impe Ministries on the front page of *The Charlotte Observer* and decided to run the program two times at their cost and pay for additional advertising.

In Greenville, South Carolina, it's even worse. The station cancelled the program two hours in advance of the airing because of 14 calls. One hundred sixty-five stations aired the program without problems. How unfair to cancel a program because of 14 protesters. A few of them said they had seen the program. Obviously, since Greenville is about 100 miles south of Charlotte, they saw only the first half of the program. In it, Bob Winter, a converted gay, tells of his conversion and asks other gays to abandon this lifestyle. How sad when freedom of speech is prohibited in order to please a minority group.

In Lansing, Michigan, the program was cancelled. In an article by Sue Nichols in the *Lansing State Journal*, I was called an alarmist. However, page 5A was very revealing as the reporter stated, "Groups advocating Gay rights expressed concern that Van Impe links a disease with a moral judgment. 'I think it does a lot of damage,' said Liz McGough, acting executive director of the Michigan Organization for Human Rights, a statewide Gay and Lesbian rights organization."

Now let's get down to basics. Am I an alarmist?

If I am, it's because of using the multiplied reports I have accumulated from the very media who now accuse me of being an alarmist. It's their stuff. Judge for yourself.

"Paranoia in the Gay community may be preventing government agencies from taking tougher action to tackle the acquired immune deficiency syndrome epidemic," according to the President's closest adviser on the disease.

"This disease has been handled unlike any other comparable situation that I can think of historically." Gary Bauer,

JVI Progress Report (October 1987).

Reagan's chief domestic policy adviser, said in an interview with *The Chronicle*, "Perhaps government at all levels hasn't done enough that prudence would have required government to do, given that some folks feel we're dealing with the equivalent of the Black Plague." (*San Francisco Chronicle*, April 30, 1987.)

Those who make it their business to worry about the disease are very worried indeed. Their concern, in blunt language, is that AIDS is on the verge of "breaking out" into the population at large.

If I am an alarmist, then read the following and thank God that I am willing to bear the brunt of warning a nation.

"Why then, have public health officials soft-pedaled their estimates? Virin, (co-chairman of the American Foundation for AIDS Research) says the reason is to [watch the wording] 'avoid alarming the public.' She adds, 'They are lulling people into complacency.'

"In 20 years, a significant portion of our society could be incapacitated. We could end up with two societies — those who have it and those who don't.

"With cases doubling every 13 months, AIDS will soon take its place in Rogue's gallery of major world scourges. The death toll could be in the tens of millions." (James Miller, *U.S. News and World Report*, January 12, 1987.)

How hypocritical the media is by classifying me as an alarmist because I believe and quote their materials.

Dr. Jack Van Impe Progress Report (October 1987).

What the Experts Are Saying About AIDS — More Alarming Announcements

AIDS will probably prove to be the plague of the millennium.

Alvin F. Kein, M.D., New York University Medical Center

Alarming AIDS Announcements

We are in the very early stage of what all evidence indicates may be a terrible world-wide epidemic, possibly killing 10 percent of the population or more. AIDS may kill 22 million Americans in the next few years. What we have to do, and quickly, is to get our people and more specifically our young people to change their sexual behavior. Promiscuity is a certain way to get infected with HTLV-III. Our young people especially need to know that sex transmits AIDS. Everyone needs to know this.

Ronald K. Wright, M.D. Chief Medical Examiner, Broward County, Florida, Associate Professor of Pathology and Epidemiology, University of Miami School of Medicine.

AIDS is a national medical disaster.

Paul Valberding, M.D., San Francisco General Hospital

In the Italian magazine *Prospective Nel Mondo*, Jesuit priest Father Sgreccia wrote that, "All the human race will be infected by AIDS in 17 years, unless emergency health measures are taken.

"The stark truth facing America, and the rest of the world, is that we are today confronted with a plague of potentially unprecedented dimensions. The death toll from AIDS could reach truly horrific figures in the not-too-distant future."

Journalist Elsie W. Graves

There will be an inexorable spread of AIDS into the heterosexual community.

William McCormack, M.D., *Sexually Transmitted Diseases*.

Anyone who has the least ability to look into the future can already see the potential for this disease being much worse than anything mankind has seen before.

Wards Cates, M.D., Centers for Disease Control

It is reasonable to assume that in many areas the number of persons infected with HTLV-III/LAV is at least one hundred times higher than that of reported cases of AIDS....

J. W. Curran, M.D., *The Epidemiology and Prevention of the Acquired Immunodeficiency Syndrome: Annals of Internal Medicine*, (Vol. 103, 1985).

The AIDS epidemic is not tapering off. At present, the Centers for Disease Control (CDC) has reported more than 35,000 cases.

Within four years, the Public Health Service predicts the number will reach 350,000. Unfortunately, those people officially diagnosed with AIDS represent only the tip of the iceberg.

Dr. James Curran of the CDC has stated, "In many areas, the number of persons infected with the AIDS virus is at least one hundred times greater than the reported cases."

In his July 22, 1985 testimony before Congress, Dr. Dani Bolognesi of the Duke University Medical Center asserted that two million Americans were already permanently infected with the AIDS virus and capable of spreading the disease.

The number of infected persons, he contended, could be "expected to double each year."

At the present, there are between three and four million infectious carriers of the AIDS virus in the United States. If each carrier establishes a "monogamous" relationship with only one other healthy person, the number of infectious car-

Drs. Redfield, Babcock, Seale

Alarming AIDS Announcements

riers will double....

Barring effective public health measures, it is conservatively estimated that by 1991 there will be 12 to 15 million infectious carriers in the United States alone.

Worldwide, Dr. Halfdahn Mahler, director of the World Health Organization, asserts that 100 million persons will be infected with AIDS by 1991.

Dr. James Slaff, former medical investigator at the National Institute of Health, has pointed out in his book, *The AIDS Epidemic*, that 30 to 45 percent of those infected with the AIDS virus develop AIDS or ARC (AIDS related complex) within five years after initial infection.

Dr. William Haseltine of Harvard states that within five to ten years the vast majority of those infected will face severe life threatening illness.

In graphic terms, over the next several years millions of Americans will have their bodies and minds devastated by the AIDS virus.

The predictions of Dr. Robert Redfield of Walter Reed Army Medical Center is that *10 million Americans may be infected by 1991*, four years away.

However, statistical expert Donald E. Babcock, Ph.D., predicts 23 million deaths within four years, 1991. The number infected but still alive could be ten times as much, or 230 million — meaning everybody.

British expert Dr. John Seale gives the human race 50 years before it becomes extinct.

Dr. Robert Redfield, Donald E. Babcock, Ph.D., Dr. John Seale

A world-wide AIDS epidemic will become so serious it will dwarf such earlier medical disasters as the Black Plague, smallpox, and typhoid. If we can't make progress, we face the dreadful prospect of a world-wide death toll in

Otis R. Bowen, Secretary, Health and Human Services

the tens of millions a decade from now.

Otis R. Bowen, Secretary, Health and Human Services

Millions to Die

Dr. Paul Kaldahl, pathologist from Oklahoma City, warned, "It has all the ear-markings of a world-wide disaster, a 20th century plague. Millions are destined to die apart from a medical miracle." No one is expecting any miracles, medical or otherwise. In fact, researchers have compared AIDS to the Bubonic Plague (Black Death) that killed one-third of the entire population of Europe — 75,000,000 people during the Middle Ages!

Dr. Paul Kaldahl, pathologist, Oklahoma City, Oklahoma

AIDS in 91 Nations

The World Health Organization (WHO), headquartered in Geneva, announced on February 13, 1987, that 91 nations have reported cases of AIDS. This is more than double the number of nations reporting such cases a year ago. Of 40,638 cases reported to WHO by February 12, 72.6 percent are from the USA.

The World Health Organization

The Big AIDS Cover-Up

The federal CDC definition of AIDS is so narrow that most who die from AIDS are not listed in AIDS statistics, but as deaths from AIDS Related Complex, ARC. The CDC keeps no statistics on ARC, even though there are 5 to 10 times as many cases of ARC as AIDS. *The Wall Street Journal* of May 30, 1986, quoted that ratio which is too low. The more reliable *Medical Laboratory Observer* magazine of November 1985, estimated that there are "10 to 20 times more people with ARC than diagnosable AIDS."

The Wall Street Journal, (May 30, 1986), and *Medical Laboratory Observer,* (November 1985).

Alarming AIDS Announcements

Worried for the World

Ursula Naccache, a senior editor in *The Digest's European Bureau*, attended an international conference on AIDS, held in Paris, and found researchers frightened by what they saw happening in Central Africa. A few weeks later at a reception in Washington, D.C., Roving Editor John Pekkanen, a prize-winning reporter and highly respected medical writer, heard an infectious-disease expert disclose, almost casually, that the AIDS epidemic had become so widespread in Central Africa he feared that region of the world was "gone."

"I had read news reports about Africa's AIDS problem," says Pekkanen, "but to hear such a respected authority speak in such bleak terms astounded me."

The extent of the epidemic was little known because many African countries had clamped a lid of secrecy on AIDS information. But we were convinced it was a story of such magnitude that it had to be told. So Pekkanen, with research help from Naccache, set out on its trail.

Pekkanen began by interviewing AIDS researchers in the United States, Great Britain, France, and Switzerland. Then he and Naccache went to Africa for three weeks of investigative reporting in five African countries. First stop was Brazzaville, Congo, where the World Health Organization (WHO) was holding the first major African conference on AIDS — and the first one there that Western journalists were allowed to attend. Only *Reader's Digest*, Radio-Canada and Britain's Independent Television News (ITN) were represented. Many Africans talked publicly about the epidemic, but there was considerable stonewalling by government officials angered by what they regarded as insulting charges that AIDS began in Africa.

Reader's Digest (June 1987).

Alarming AIDS Announcements

Pekkanen prefers on-the-record interviews. But he soon learned if he insisted on this, he would get very little useful information. So Pekkenen and Naccache promised anonymity to most of the African AIDS experts they interviewed. It was then that these men and women, many of them physicians, dropped their official facade and confided to the *Reader's Digest* team how devastating they felt the AIDS epidemic had become. Many expressed a profound grief in private that contrasted sharply with their public postures.

"I remember talking to a Ugandan physician, a man of high intelligence and great humor," Pekkanen says. "I asked him if he was worried for his country. He looked at me and said, 'I am worried for the world.' "

Reader's Digest: Behind the Lines, (June 1987).

Deathwatch Over Haiti
Doctors Fear 1 in 19 May Carry AIDS

PORT-AU-PRINCE, Haiti — Crippled by poverty, dangerously overpopulated, and struggling to find a new political identity, the small country of Haiti faces yet another disaster: a growing epidemic of AIDS that threatens to wipe out its healthiest young workers.

As many as one in 10 residents of this capital city may carry the virus that causes AIDS, and doctors fear the infection is seeping out into remote rural areas where it will be virtually impossible to detect, control, or treat.

Ellen Hale, *Gannett News Service*

How AIDS Could Wipe Out All Americans in Six to Seven Years

The deadly pandemic AIDS, for which there is no known cure, is currently spreading at such an alarming rate that the

National Democratic Policy Committee (October 1985).

Alarming AIDS Announcements

number of confirmed victims of the disease, according to medical experts, is doubling every six months. What does this mean for the United States? When a deadly pandemic doubles its victims every six months, how fast is it growing?

Below is a stark calculation of how fast a doubling rate is. The calculation in the left-hand column is based on the Atlanta Centers for Disease Control (CDC) "official" estimates of confirmed cases, which they reported to be approximately 12,000 last June (now, nearly 14,000). The calculation in the right-hand column is based on the more probable situation. Medical and health professionals generally agree that the CDC figures are vastly underestimated. "Official" estimates are that as many as 1.5 million Americans are carrying AIDS antibodies, indicating that they have been "infected" with the disease, even though they may not yet be suffering from the disease itself.

How AIDS Could Destroy America

THE AIDS DOUBLING RATE

Date	CDC Estimate No. of victims	More Probable Medical Estimate No. of victims
June 1985	12,000 cases	100,000 cases
Jan. 1986	24,000	200,000
June	48,000	400,000
Jan. 1987	96,000	800,000
June	192,000	1,600,000
Jan. 1988	384,000	3,200,000
June	768,000	6,400,000
Jan. 1989	1,500,000	12,800,000
June	3,000,000	25,600,000
Jan. 1990	6,000,000	51,000,000
June	12,000,000	102,000,000
Jan. 1991	24,000,000	204,000,000
June	48,000,000	No Americans left!
Jan. 1992	96,000,000	No Americans left!
June	192,000,000	No Americans left!
Jan. 1993	No Americans left!	

Alarming AIDS Announcements

One leading medical school on the West Coast has published a study which shows that the actual number of AIDS victims is from 3 to 10 times higher than the CDC "official" statistics. That would mean that, in reality, at least 140,000 Americans may already be AIDS victims, and 14 million may be walking around with the antibodies indicating that they have been exposed to the disease.

The projections in the chart are based on two startling estimates. The left-hand column is based on the underestimated "official" CDC statistics. The right-hand column is based on the more probable figures reported by medical and public health officials around the country.

Thus, without a crash effort, even the conservative figures in the left-hand column indicate that the U.S. population would be wiped out at some time between June 1992 and January 1993. The more probable figures on the right (which themselves are, most likely, conservative) indicate an endpoint between January and June of 1991. In short, if the doubling rate continues, and does not accelerate, the U.S. population has between six and eight years before every American could be infected by a disease which kills everyone who gets it!

. The designation "No Americans Left" in the chart indicates that, at that point, the number of victims caused by the AIDS doubling rate will have exceeded the total U.S. population.

But will the disease always continue to double every six months? Not necessarily. There are two possibilities, and only two possibilities:

1) The disease rate will accelerate, and take off even faster than doubling every six months. It could suddenly spread in non-linear fashion at an even faster rate, with one deadly disease "piggybacking" upon

National Democratic Policy Committee (October 1985).

another, as they recombine into ever more deadly strains. This, of course, would bring closer the point at which the disease infects everybody.

2) The AIDS doubling rate will be halted by the nation imposing traditional emergency Public Health Measures. Throughout history, pandemics have not been stopped by "miracle cures," but by the society imposing strict Public Health Measures to stop the contagion from spreading. If the disease is contained, then medical research — if adequately funded — has the time to make research breakthroughs.

National Democratic Policy Committee (October 1985).

Blood Transfusion for Woman
Was Fatal Dose of AIDS

A doctor walked into the suburban San Francisco hospital waiting room where Bob Borchelt and his four children waited for news of his wife Frances' hip replacement operation. The doctor called the surgery a success.

The family was relieved. Nobody could remember the last time Frances was ever sick with anything, but she was a 71-year-old woman, and any surgery, however routine, could be risky.

A few days later, Frances Borchelt was her feisty self and fell into a fierce argument with a niece. A doctor had wanted to give her a blood transfusion, she complained.

"I told them I don't want one," she said.

Frances did not know that loss of blood during her surgery had required the transfusion of two pints of blood. A third unit, doctors said, was transfused as a precaution. The third unit had been donated by a young man two weeks before — a man who did not fill out his donor referral card properly.

Frances Borchelt was released from Seton Medical Center in San Francisco on August 30, but she still had not regained her strength. She was weak, running continuous, unexplained fevers.

She was released from the hospital with a temperature of 100 degrees. Once home, she was so fatigued that she was incapable of performing the exercises necessary to gain use of her new hip.

It was during this time that the bill for Frances' operation arrived from the hospital. Because Medicare did not pay for blood transfusions, the cost of three units of blood from Irwin Memorial Blood Bank was included on the invoice.

Shilts, *And the Band Played On* (1987).

Blood

That was how the Borchelt family learned about Frances' blood transfusion.

In the six months since Frances had been given the transfusion, she had not regained her health. Her fatigue was so relentless that she could no longer bustle through the busy days that had characterized her life.

In early February, the nightmare turned darker. It started with a psoriasis rash on Frances' arms. Before long, the itchy red rash covered her body, from the top of her scalp to the soles of her feet.

By September 1984 — more than a year after her hip replacement surgery — Frances still had not recovered. The painful psoriasis persisted; she had not regained the 20 pounds lost during her bout with hepatitis.

In August, a case of the sniffles turned into a cold that would not go away. Frances either trembled from chills or sweated profusely from fevers that peaked daily at 103 degrees. As usual, the doctors were baffled.

Sometimes Frances asked her husband, Bob, to hold her. Even as he became drenched in her sweat, Bob stared down on his suffering wife, feeling pity and compassion and sorrow, wishing desperately that he could do something to ease her agony.

One doctor suggested Frances was suffering from psitacosis when they admitted her to the hospital this time. Maybe she had picked up the disease from the family parakeet, he said. Frances' daughter, Cathy had studied AIDS brochures and believed her mother had AIDS, but the doctors were adamant that she did not have any of the symptoms.

They cultured Frances' blood, tested her bone marrow, and used every gadget of nuclear medicine to see what was wrong. Meanwhile, she grew weaker with each passing day.

Shilts, *And the Band Played On* (1987).

Breathing was becoming excruciatingly difficult.

Cathy was at work in the San Francisco Police Department's record room when a co-worker handed her the morning paper and asked about the story on page eight. It was an announcement by the Irwin Memorial Blood Bank that an ailing, unnamed woman at Seton Medical Center had contracted AIDS through blood provided by Irwin in August 1983.

"Is that your mom?"

It was the first time anybody in the Borchelt family was informed that Frances was indeed suffering from transfusion-associated AIDS.

That evening at the hospital, Cathy was watching television with her mother when the newscaster began talking about the new transfusion case in Seton Medical Center. Frances shook her head sadly at the news.

"That poor lady," she said. "If it were me, I'd sue."

Cathy was shocked. Obviously, nobody had told her mother yet that she had AIDS. That night, Bob Borchelt insisted that the doctors tell Frances what had happened.

May 17, 1985

Throughout the last weeks of May, it seemed there was no end to the litany of ailments that struck Frances. She had severe lymphadenopathy, and the doctors had now diagnosed a blood disease, idiopathic thrombocytopenic purpura, as well. She also had mastitis and oral thrush.

Frances tried to act as if she could live a normal life. Every morning, she made her bed, as she had always done during her four decades of marriage. Now, however, tidying the sheets sometimes took 45 minutes; she just didn't have the energy.

On Monday, June 10, 1985, the family took Frances back to Seton Medical Center to be treated for bronchial pneu-

Shilts, *And the Band Played On* (1987).

Blood

monia. Her lungs filled with fluids, and she sweated continuously from fierce fevers.

On Saturday, June 15 Frances went blind.

Frances had been adamant that she did not want to be buried with her wedding rings. As her body began to fill with fluids and bloat, Cathy decided it was time to remove them.

Bob sat with his wife all day on Monday, June 17. She had drifted into a deeper coma, and the nurses, seeing Bob's exhaustion, suggested that he go home and rest. They'd phone him if anything happened.

The call came not long after Bob got back home. Frances was dead.

Randy Shilts, *And the Band Played On*: "Politics, People, and the AIDS Epidemic" (Copyright © 1987 by Randy Shilts, St. Martin's Press, Inc., New York).

Ten-year Risk Factor

Persons who have engaged in homosexual activities or have shot street drugs within the last ten years should never donate blood.

Surgeon General Koop's Report

Homo Sells Tainted Blood

Joseph Edward Markowski, 29,...admitted he sold blood for $8 a pint knowing he might spread AIDS...

"I know that AIDS can kill. But I was so hard up for money I didn't give a _____," district attorney Ira Reiner quoted Markowski as saying.

Markowski also gave investigators names of five male sex clients.

News Record: "Investigators Seeking Blood of AIDS Donor" (Associated Press, June 30, 1987), p. 3.

Red Cross Brochure

Front Page of a Red Cross Brochure: What You Must Know Before Giving Blood

If you are a man who has had sex with another man since 1977, you must not give blood or plasma.

(THIS MESSAGE APPEARS ON THE REVERSE SIDE OF BROCHURE)

Thank You for Coming in Today

Please read this pamphlet carefully before you agree to give blood or plasma. You will be asked to sign a statement that says you have read this information today, that you understand it, and that if you are at risk for spreading the AIDS virus, you will not give blood or plasma for transfusion to another person.

Your Safety

To be sure you can give blood or plasma safely today, we will take your blood pressure, pulse, and temperature. A drop of blood from your finger or ear lobe will be tested to make sure that giving a pint of blood will not make you anemic. We will also ask you questions about your health.

If you can donate, a Red Cross worker will use a new, sterile needle to take about one pint of blood or plasma from a vein in your arm. The needle will be discarded when you are finished donating. You cannot get AIDS or any infectious disease by donating blood or plasma.

Patient Safety

The blood or plasma you donate will be given to sick people. If any of the information in the next section applies to you, do not give blood or plasma, because it might harm a

Red Cross Brochure

Blood

patient who receives it.

AIDS is a disease that breaks down the body's system for fighting infection and disease. AIDS can be spread through donated blood and plasma. Blood tests to detect antibody [sic] to the AIDS virus (HTLV-III) are very good, but they are *not* perfect. *It is possible for a person in the early stage of infection to have a negative test result.* Therefore, people who are at risk for getting AIDS must never give blood or plasma.

Red Cross Brochure

One Small Virion

...The amount of blood dried on a needle is miniscule, but that is all it takes to get AIDS.

Dr. James McKeever, Ph.D., *The AIDS Plague*, p. 62-64.

Here is an example from 20/20 of how tainted plasma was handled:

If we can't trust the plasma donor, can we trust the collector?...To assure safety, collected plasma is first stored in a freezer. It's not supposed to be shipped out to a processor until the results are back from the lab. Should any of the plasma test positive for AIDS or hepatitis, it's called a hot unit, marked "reactive" and destroyed. Or at least that's what's supposed to happen. [on camera] This is a letter for the FDA suspending a Michigan plasma center's license last June. The offense: shipping plasma positive for both hepatitis and AIDS. There were other offenses, and the list goes on...

Tom Jarriel, *20/20-ABC News Transcripts*: "Blood When You Have No Choice" (March 19, 1987), p. 10.

One Unit in 20,000 Units Dangerous

The inclusion of one unit of plasma in a pool of up to 20,000 units from a person who later developed AIDS and whose plasma at the time of donation may be been infectious, could have a profound effect...

John C. Petricciani, M.D., *Annals of Internal Medicine*: "Licensed Tests for Antibody to Human T-Lymphotropic Virus Type III" (1985), Vol. 103.

Deadly Errors in Present Tests

It won't be long before the public learns that the highly touted *AIDS-antibody test is chock-full of error* — both false-positive and false-negatives — and therefore carries no guarantee of an AIDS-free national blood supply.

Dr. Robert Mendelsohn, *Newsletter*: "Special Report: AIDS" (Noebel/Lutton/Cameron, November 10, 1985), Vol. 9, p. 2.

No Fool-proof Tests

No fool-proof blood-screening test currently exists to protect our population against AIDS. A blood test exists that will detect the existence of antibodies to HTLV-III. But some persons infected with HTLV-III do not produce antibodies to AIDS and have no current symptoms of AIDS.

Review of the Public Health Service's Response to AIDS, a Report issued by the Office of Technology Assessment.

Transmission

It is now known that blood used for transfusions is being screened for antibody to the virus. There have been cases where persons have been tested and found to be negative for the antibody and yet positive for the virus. The blood from such persons would therefore, not be identified by the present antibody screening test and could normally be available for transfusion.

Charles Marwick, *JAMA — (Journal of the American Medical Association)*: "AIDS-associated Virus Yields Data to Intensify in Scientific Study" (November 22-29, 1985), Vol. 254, No. 20.

Blood

Devastating Findings

With public-health officials and politicians thrashing out who should be tested for infection with the AIDS virus and how the test results should be used, the accuracy of the test itself has been nearly ignored.

But last month, a study by Congress' Office of Technology Assessment broke this drought of information. Using data from the College of American Pathologists, the study found that *the tests can be very inaccurate indeed*...For high-risk people...the test produces false negatives about 10 percent of the time, meaning that 1 in 10 of these people are told they're not infected when they are. The main reason for the inaccuracies, the OTA found, was that many labs perform the Western blot — the second of the two tests routinely used to detect AIDS infection — very poorly. Says the OTA's Dr. Larry Miike, who conducted the study, "Many labs are doing a good job, and a few bad labs may be causing the problem."

Because some seven percent of the U.S. population has gotten the test, the study suggests that hundreds of people, possibly thousands...think they're not infected when they are. Says Dr. Mervyn Silverman, president of the American Foundation for AIDS Research, "These mistakes can have devastating emotional and public-health consequences. Large state-run and accredited labs that do thousands of the tests are very reliable. Even so, health officials say the OTA study strengthens the argument against mass, mandatory AIDS screening, because of the risk of error....

U.S. News & World Report (Copyright, November 23, 1987). Used by permission.

Disturbing News About AIDS-virus Test A Fever Lurking in the Blood
Latest Findings From Finland — Tests Take One Full Year

Growing numbers of Americans have been having their blood tested, hoping for assurance that they don't carry the deadly AIDS virus. Now comes a jolt of bad news: Some of the people given a clean bill of health may in fact be harboring the virus after all. Scientists reached that conclusion recently when a new study from Finland found that the virus at times remains unnoticed by the conventional tests until it has been in the system for a year or more.

The test now in use, which identifies antibodies to the AIDS virus, was thought to pick up infection within six to 12 weeks. By suggesting that the danger period extends to more than a year, the research indicates that to be truly safe, people need to take a series of tests and steel themselves for a much longer time of anxiety....

U.S. News & World Report (Copyright, October 12, 1987).Used by permission.

AIDS Virus Can Go Undetected for Up to 14 Months

WASHINGTON — A person may be infected with the AIDS virus for up to 14 months without the virus being detected by tests for AIDS antibodies, much longer than previously thought, according to a published report.

Scientists had previously thought that antibodies to the virus usually develop between three weeks and 12 weeks after infection, *The Washington Post* noted in its Friday editions.

The newspaper reported on a study of sexually active gay men by researchers from the National Cancer Institute in

Associated Press (October 1987).

Finland. The study was published in the British medical journal *The Lancet*, the newspaper said, but the date of the issue was not given.

"The results surprised us," National Cancer Institute researcher Genoveffa Franchini, an author of the study told the newspaper. "What it means is clear.

"The period before the development of antibodies is longer than anyone thought. But we still don't know how long people are infected with this disease before it appears on tests."

The *Post* said the study suggests that negative test results for thousands of people who have taken the AIDS-antibody test in the last two years may have been premature...

In the new study, researchers used an antigen test that can detect several proteins made by the AIDS virus and identified the very beginning of the infection as many as fourteen months before the men showed antibodies to HIV.

"There are many unanswered questions," Franchini said. "We don't know how many sexual contacts these people have had, and we don't know what other factors could have contributed to their infection."

She said it is important to develop a test to measure how much virus is needed to infect cells.

"The implications are still uncertain," she said. "We just don't know where it will lead yet."

The Associated Press (October 1987).

Three New Strains of Deadly Virus

There's been at least two or three completely new strains of AIDS for which the ELISA test is not even effective...we may have a virus being spread at the present time just as AIDS was spread in the early days before we knew that it existed, undetected and a virus which could be introduced

Drs. Mark, Rowe, AIDS Prevention Institute.

into our blood transfusions would be a dangerous thing and people, the general members of our population who are not sexually promiscuous and who are not drug addicts, may get a very unfortunate virus injected into their system even quite unwittingly, quite innocently.

Dr. Vernon A. Mark, Associate Professor of Surgery, New National AIDS Prevention Institute: (Harvard Medical School: Interview with Dr. Ed Rowe, President, March 1987).

New Strain Undetected by Tests

Another alarming development is the recent discovery of a new strain of the AIDS virus that has gone undetected by standard blood tests. According to French Dr. Luc Montaigner of the Pasteur Institute, "This is bad news for blood banks." An estimated 30,000 Americans have already been infected with AIDS as a result of contaminated blood transfusions. *The non-detection of this new strain and the failure to include AIDS dementia in the current figures show that the situation is far worse than it appears.*

Albert Veldhuyzen, *CWA Newsletter:* "The Problems With the Surgeon General's Report on AIDS" (May 1987), Vol. 9 No. 5.

Stick With Trusted Friends

After sitting through the meeting [an advisory committee meeting convened by the CDC], one observer said, "I know what I'd do if I were going to have elective surgery. I'd get all my friends and relatives to donate blood for me."

William A. Check, Ph.D., *JAMA — (Journal of the American Medical Association):* "Preventing AIDS Transmission: Should Blood Donors Be Screened?" (1983), Vol. 249.

Transmission:
Store Up Personal Blood

Apparently the American Medical Association is becoming alarmed because on November 6, 1986, the AMA

Courtney, *The Independent American* (February 1987).

Blood

recommended that people anticipating elective heart, chest, or orthopedic surgery have their own blood collected in a six-week period before the operation. The method, called autologous blood transfusion, eliminates the risk of contracting AIDS or other communicable diseases associated with receiving someone else's blood, said Dr. Ira Friedlander, a member of the AMA's Council on Scientific Affairs.

Phoebe Courtney, *The Independent American*: "Can AIDS Threaten You?" (February 1987), No. 217.

AIDS: What Do We Do Now?

(An interview with American Red Cross president Richard Schubert.)

1. **Why will AIDS spread so fast?**
   Because we can't convince enough people to modify their life style. Right now there are between one-and-a-half million and two million carriers, and fewer than 50,000 of them know it. The rest are doing their thing and infecting others.

2. **Does the medical community know more than it's telling because they're afraid to say what's really spreading AIDS?**
   Not that I can tell. Here at the Red Cross we stay very close to scientists and the Centers for Disease Control. They honestly do not know a great deal...

3. **So if my 12-year-old daughter gets hit by a car and needs three pints of blood, you can assure me there's nothing to fear?**
   No, I can't promise you that — but I couldn't before AIDS came along either. Donated blood has never been totally safe. That's why we, as an institution, say

Christian Herald Magazine (January 1988).

transfusions are only for compelling need. We've always encouraged pre-deposit — where if you know you're going to need surgery, you put your own blood aside in advance.

We do have one small problem: There's a time lag after infection with the AIDS virus before the person's system creates antibodies, which is what shows up in a blood test. So if the blood donor just got AIDS and then gave blood, it's possible we might not screen it. But chances of that happening are very small these days, because we're asking all blood donors a lot of questions, giving them three and four chances to say quietly, "Well, maybe you'd better not use my blood."

4. **What if somebody with AIDS were on the kitchen crew for a church potluck supper? Would you think twice about going through the line?**
I might think twice about it...but hopefully I'd be responsible, not irrational and operating on phobias. Remember the sparrow; trust the good Lord to take care of you.

5. **Should we worry about an AIDS baby in the church nursery?**
No, subject to normal precautions. Now if that baby falls and begins to bleed, the workers should take precautions, since blood is a transmitter of AIDS. But that doesn't mean you have to clear out the nursery or day care center.

6. **We face more than 270,000 AIDS cases and more than 179,000 deaths between now and 1991...**
— Excuse me; some people think those numbers are quite low.

7. **...But 500,000 people die each year from heart attacks. Why is AIDS so much more important than**

Christian Herald Magazine (January 1988).

heart attacks, which will kill far more people between now and 1991?

Heart attacks fall predominantly among older people, and the victim often survives. AIDS focuses on the young (primarily because of their life-style), and it's 100 percent fatal.

Another thing: Heart attacks are not communicable. AIDS is.

Did You Know?

Before AIDS, there were only three known lentiviruses, also incurable. They were confined to sheep, horses, and goats. Infected animals were slaughtered to stop the spread.

Richard Schubert, President, American Red Cross, *Christian Herald* Magazine (January 1988).

Doctors Told To Be Careful AIDS Is Easier To Catch Than Imagined
Hospital Group Sets AIDS Guidelines

More than 100,000 Michigan medical workers come under new anti-AIDS guidelines that call for wearing protective gear — including gloves, goggles, masks, and gowns — when there's a chance of being exposed to a patient's blood or other fluids.

Thousands of patients, even those who don't have AIDS, would be treated by gear-wearing nurses and doctors, under recommendations issued by the American Hospital Association at a national meeting last week in Atlanta.

Patients without AIDS would be treated as if they had an infectious disease, creating a policy of "universal precaution."

A Michigan doctor attending the Atlanta meeting admitted he no longer performs mouth-to-mouth resuscitation in the hospital because of his fear of AIDS.

"I consider that an unfair risk to myself and my family," said Dr. Gregory Henry, director of the emergency department at Beyer Memorial Hospital in Ypsilanti.

"We are coming into a whole new world," he said. "I know of no resident who hasn't stuck himself with a needle or cut himself before his training is over. It's part of the learning experience. But now there may be a much higher price for that education."

Dr. Richard Yerian, chief medical consultant of the health facilities bureau at the state health department, estimated that 15,000 residents would test positive for the AIDS virus "and for the most part they have no idea they are infected."

Jeff Keeton, president of the Detroit Emergency Medical Service (EMS) union that represents 180 technicians and

Angell, *The Detroit News* (August 2, 1987).

paramedics, said he is setting up a seminar on the issue, and contract negotiators are discussing the problem with the city.

"When you roll up where someone is bleeding, you have no idea that the person has AIDS," Keeton said.

Although EMS technicians have disposable gloves, Keeton wants them also to have eye goggles, masks, and gowns. In addition, he wants some method where EMS technicians are told by a hospital if a patient has AIDS.

Keeton said he personally has treated four persons who had AIDS. The first time occurred six months ago.

The man told Keeton that he had AIDS. "My reaction? This could cost me my life. All kinds of things ran through my head, like you like to help people but is this worth it?"

"The underlying message to hospitals," said Margaret Domanski, director of social work and discharge planning at Ford, "is to realize that AIDS is here to stay and they/we need our staff to be prepared clinically and attitudinally to care for the persons with AIDS."

The federal Centers for Disease Control reported that nine health workers had been infected with the AIDS virus. *Four persons were infected by needle pricks, two by extensive contact with body fluids of an infected patient, and three from brief skin exposure to AIDS-contaminated blood.*

Of the skin exposure cases, one health care worker had badly chapped hands, a second had dermatitis on one ear, and the third was splashed with large amounts of blood from a collection device and was not wearing goggles.

Dwight E. M. Angell, *The Detroit News* (August 2, 1987). Reprinted with permission of *The Detroit News*, a Gannett newspaper, copyright 1987.

Virtually Safe? Bodily Fluids

The August 23, 1985, issue of the *Indianapolis Star* reported that "specialists said Thursday it is virtually

Drs. Gallo, Groopman, Haseltine

impossible to catch the disease from mosquito bites or ordinary day-to-day activities such as shaking hands."

Notice the word, "virtually." The "experts" always qualify their statements with ambiguities such as "usually," "most of the time," and "virtually." Saying you are "virtually" safe from getting AIDS through casual contact is like saying that the daring acrobat "virtually" caught the trapeze; however, he really fell and broke his sincere neck!

The "experts" give me no assurances at all with their pompous declarations. Let them tell the 5 percent (or more) of AIDS victims who have no idea how they contracted AIDS that they are "virtually" safe.

But it gets worse. According to Dr. Robert Gallo in *Lancet*, a British medical journal, December 22-29, 1985, issue, there is evidence to suggest that the AIDS virus can be transmitted through saliva.

This research seems to have been supported by that of Dr. Jerome E. Groopman of New England Deaconess Hospital as reported in the February 12, 1986 issue of the *The Indianapolis Star*. Dr. Groopman has found the AIDS virus in the saliva of 44 percent of the victims of a pre-AIDS syndrome called AIDS-Related Complex, or ARC. So we have the AIDS virus in blood, semen, saliva, mother's milk — what next?

How about sweat? Harvard pathologist William Haseltine is quoted in the *Conservative Digest*, the December 1985 issue, as saying, "Nobody can give you an absolute guarantee that one out of a hundred thousand times someone isn't going to transmit it (AIDS-causing virus) on a drinking glass or through sweat. All we can say, and all we should say, is that so far, to our knowledge, it hasn't happened." Yet!

Dr. Robert Gallo, Dr. Jerome E. Groopman, Dr. William Haseltine

Casual Contact

Fluids Splashed on Face

Dear Dr. Van Impe,

I thoroughly enjoyed and totally agreed with you on your sermon on AIDS.

As a laboratory technologist at Henry Ford Hospital working in the Serology Department, I perform the HIV antibody test and see a high rate of reactive serum specimens. The epidemic is now being evidenced in large cities soon to reach and effect small communities like Clarkston, Mich.

I had an unfortunate accident while working in the Virology Department, processing and transferring blood from an AIDS patient. The vacutainer tube broke in my hands and splashed all over the front of my lab coat, shirt and two drops fell onto my face right next to my eye. I washed my face immediately and changed clothing. A doctor from Infectious Disease Clinic was called in and spoke to me. He said since the blood only had skin contact and not mucous membrane contact I was probably at no risk of contracting the disease. He said I had an option of either doing nothing or being tested and monitored for HIV antibody and T4/T8 ratio. I believe that God does not want to take me out of His service by this disease originating from sexual perverts. I thanked God that the accident was not worse than it was.

— R. R., Clarkston, MI

Catching AIDS From Symptomless Carriers

Meanwhile, the 1.5 million to 4 million Americans who are carrying the killer virus without symptoms are unwittingly but unquestionably passing it on to many millions more.

J. Carry, B. Quick, R. Riley, *U.S. News & World Report*: "AIDS: A Time of Testing" (April 20, 1987).

Infected for Life

Dr. William Haseltine of Boston's Dana-Farley Cancer Institute says, "Once infected, a person is infected for the rest of his life. Once infected, a person is infectious. It's not safe to assume otherwise."

M. Clark, M. Gosnell, D. Witherspoon, M. Hager, V. Coppola *Newsweek*: "AIDS" (August 12, 1985).

Little Hope for the Infected

On the basis of present knowledge, we have no choice but to assume that the majority of infected persons will actually come down with the disease. (Dr. Sonigo, researcher with the Yves Montaigner group, Pasteur Institute in Paris).

Dr. Jonathan Tennenbaum, *Executive Intelligence Review*: "Medical Experts Warn of a 'Breakout' of AIDS Disease" (October 4, 1985).

Frequent Exposure Is Risky Business

Dr. Anthony S. Fauci, director of the National Institute of Allergy and Infectious Diseases (which also is at the National Institutes of Health): "There's indirect evidence to suggest that, when a person is frequently exposed to someone who is virus-positive, then there's a greater chance of that person getting infected..."

Charles Marwick, *JAMA — (Journal of the American Medical Association)*: "AIDS-associated Virus Yields Data to Intensifying Scientific Study" (1985), Vol. 254, No. 20.

Six Percent of Cases a Mystery

Dr. Fauci contends: "The mechanisms by which the disease is transmitted are very clear. One is sexual, predominantly homosexual contact in this country. This accounts for almost three-quarters of the reported cases. The next largest group is intravenous drug abusers, who account for 17% of cases."

Marwick, *JAMA,* Vol. 254 (1985).

Casual Contact

Finally, about 6% of the adult cases of AIDS and, ... about 6% of the cases in children occur in persons who do not fall into any of the known risk groups.

Charles Marwick, *JAMA-(Journal of the American Medical Association)*: "AIDS-associated Virus Yields Data to Intensifying Scientific Study" (November 22-29, 1985), Vol. 254, No. 20.

AIDS Infects Three Health Workers: Cases Develop After Skin Is Exposed to Blood From Patients

WASHINGTON — Federal health officials said Tuesday that they have learned of three cases in which health-care workers became infected with the AIDS virus after their skin was briefly exposed to blood from infected patients.

Officials said this was the first documented spread of the AIDS virus to health workers that did not involve direct injection of infected blood into the body or prolonged exposure to body fluids. The six previously reported cases among health workers involved injection or prolonged exposure.

Federal health officials said there was no evidence that the AIDS virus passes directly through intact skin. They said each of the three workers described Tuesday had small breaks or other abnormalities in the skin through which the virus might have passed. *One also was splashed with infected blood in the mouth, where the virus might have passed through mucous membrane.*

Dr. James M. Hughes of the national Centers for Disease Control said the new cases underlined the need for strict adherence to federal guidelines for preventing healthcare workers from becoming infected with the AIDS virus.

Officials with the Centers for Disease Control, part of the U.S. Public Health Service, last week summoned 15 to 20 representatives of medical organizations to the CDC's Atlanta headquarters to discuss the new cases. Several

New York Times (1987).

people who attended the May 13 meeting said they had been instructed by federal officials not to discuss it.

AIDS Protection League

Sometime during the next century, historians will observe that the AIDS disease enjoyed extraordinary rhetorical protection as our current century wound down.

The New York Times reported recently that a case of non-sexual transmission of AIDS was made public in a "tightly controlled announcement by the Department of Health and Human Services." Other *"federal health officials said they had been ordered not to speak with the press.* Dr. William Blattner, an epidemiologist at the National Cancer Institute who is investigating the incident declined to comment."

When was the last time that scientific facts were actively suppressed by government authority? Galileo!

We taxpayers are paying the salaries and paying for the research of these officials and scientists who "decline comment."

When Rock Hudson left the best AIDS clinic in the world, in Paris, *everything he had touched was burned.*

The fact of the matter is that no scientist knows the limits of how AIDS is transmitted. But the fakery goes on, the false reassurances, in the interest of protecting a political and cultural investment in the sexual revolution.

Is it not time for a real scientist to stand up and say, "We just don't know what we are dealing with here"?

Jeffrey Hart, *Phoenix Gazette* (October 13) p. A-11.

Casual Contact

AIDS Fears Grow From Confusion —
At Risk for Ten Years After Having Sex
With Carrier of AIDS

As AIDS continues to spread, mounting fear has been matched by persistent confusion over how the virus that causes the disease is transmitted.

More than 30,000 cases of acquired immune deficiency syndrome have been reported in the United States since 1981, when the disease was first identified. More than half the patients have died. Most victims in this country have been homosexual men and intravenous drug abusers.

Four percent of cases have been attributed to the spread of the virus through heterosexual intercourse with a member of the known high-risk groups: bisexual men, drug abusers or those infected by contaminated transfusions or blood products. An unknown share of the additional three percent of cases with undetermined causes may have spread through heterosexual intercourse as well.

Part of the mystery and fear arises from the fact that many carriers of the virus are not aware of it. The virus can lurk in the body without causing diseases, and the average time between infection and diagnosis may be five years or more.

Experts estimate that up to 1.5 million Americans now are infected. A small, perhaps growing, portion are men or women infected through heterosexual intercourse with a drug user or bisexual man. Each infected person is presumed to be capable of spreading the virus to others through sexual intercourse or through blood, as in sharing contaminated needles.

Anyone who has had sexual relations with a homosexual or bisexual man in the last decade, or who had used an

Altman, *Detroit Free Press* (February 17, 1987).

unsterile needle to take drugs in the same period, is at risk of infection.

While much remains to be learned, scientists say that studies of victims and disease patterns have provided a clear picture of how the virus has spread in this country, and how it has not.

Here are some things they know:

How does AIDS spread?

Many studies have documented the spread of the AIDS virus to an uninfected person through anal or vaginal intercourse with an infected person; through exchanges of blood, such as on contaminated hypodermic needles; from infected mothers to their infants before or during birth, and possibly through breast-feeding of infants.

How can a person tell if he or she is infected with the AIDS virus?

The blood test for AIDS infection detects the presence of AIDS virus antibodies, substances the body produces in response to invasion by virus. Those who fear they may be infected can get the blood test through a personal doctor or through anonymous testing centers in many cities throughout the country.

Are some types of sexual intercourse more dangerous than others?

Many experts believe the AIDS virus spreads more readily in anal intercourse than in vaginal intercourse because anal sex often involves breaks in rectal tissues, thus allowing easier entry of the virus into the bloodstream. Studies suggest that the receptive partner in anal sex is at greater risk. One study has suggested that the virus may be able to directly infect cells in the colon.

Can the virus spread from an infected person in vaginal intercourse?

Altman, *Detroit Free Press* (February 17, 1987).

Casual Contact

Several studies clearly have shown that it can, and that it can spread both from a man to a woman and from a woman to a man in intercourse. Some experts believe transmission occurs far less often from a woman to a man than from a man to a woman, but this point is debated. *The virus has been found both in semen and in vaginal secretions of infected people.*

How is the virus transmitted in vaginal intercourse?

Scientists aren't certain. One theory is that the virus passes through invisible breaks in the surface inside the vagina or on the penis. Some experts believe the virus also may enter through mucous membranes or other soft tissues in the genital areas. No one knows if the virus can penetrate the lining of the male urethra.

What is the risk of spreading the virus from a single act of vaginal intercourse with an infected person?

Precise data are lacking. From indirect evidence, scientists judge the risk of transmission in a single encounter to be low. Quantification is complex: Some infected people have said that they had only a single exposure, while other people who have had hundreds of exposures escaped infection. *Several studies have shown that with repeated intercourse over time, as many as half the sexual partners of infected men or women become infected.*

In Africa, where vaginal intercourse is believed to be the major means of spreading AIDS, studies suggest that the virus may pass more easily among people who have had gonorrhea, genital herpes or other sexually transmitted diseases, perhaps as a result of open sores in the skin of the genital area and the presence there of larger than usual numbers of the types of white blood cells that the virus invades.

Can the virus spread through oral sex?

Federal epidemiologists suspect that it can because the

Altman, *Detroit Free Press* (February 17, 1987).

virus is present in semen and vaginal secretions and thus might enter the cells of the body through cuts or mucous membranes in the mouth or throat. However, they have not documented any such cases.

Is it dangerous to kiss an infected person?

Minute amounts of the AIDS virus have been found in the saliva of some virus carriers, but no cases of transmission by kissing have been documented. Experts say there is no danger in a peck on the cheek of an infected person but they recommend against any exchange of saliva and deep kissing with an infected person.

Is there greater likelihood of viral spread when a woman is menstruating?

No data exist [sic] on this point, but some experts suspect that it is so.

Why has AIDS spread among drug addicts?

When intravenous drug users share unsterile needles and equipment, traces of blood contaminated with the virus may be injected into the bloodstream of subsequent users of the same needle. Experts consider repeated exposure to the virus through shared needles particularly dangerous.

Can human bites transmit AIDS?

Experts believe it is theoretically possible, but know of no cases.

Can the virus be spread by insects?

Several studies in Africa and the United States have found no evidence that the virus has been spread by mosquitoes or other insects. Some laboratory studies have suggested the virus can survive in insects such as bed bugs, but studies of transmission patterns have not detected any cases spread by blood-sucking insects.

Lawrence K. Altman, *Detroit Free Press*: (Copyright © 1987, *New York Times Company*, February 17, 1987). Reprinted by permission.

Casual Contact

Note: The following information will be alphabetized under the heading of "Casual Contact" for simplification purposes. Then, after completing this section, we will return to the original plan by returning to the letter "C" and the subject of condoms.

The following facts are disputed by a few medical practitioners. Upon reaching the disinformation section of this book, it will become obvious that unreliable, distorted error by gay-pressured medical and media personnel is the cause of much of the present confusion. — JVI

Barbers

ALBANY, Georgia — Barber shaves in Georgia may go the way of the two-bit haircut. Fearing AIDS, some barbers want a state ban on razors. They said modern electric clippers eliminate the need for shaving the back of necks.

USA Today (September 28, 1987).

Barbers are humorously called "tonsorial artists." The news release above proves that AIDS is no laughing matter to these professionals. Should they nick a customer whose blood contains the deadly virus and the minutest virion enters a cut, rash, or sore they might have, it could be devastating for them. Furthermore, since the virus can live in a dried out condition for numerous days, the infected razor might become lethal to the one who hears the word "next." Should that infected blade nick one or be drawn over an existing cut, rash or sore, it could become the beginning of the end. (See Dried Virus section.)

Boxers Use AIDS Education To Reach Those at Risk

The boxers weren't the only men in the ring with gloves on

USA Today (September 28, 1987).

when heavyweight champ Mike Tyson beat up challenger Tyrell Biggs.

The trainers wore gloves. So did the referee. But the gloves were transparent rubber ones "to enhance hygienic conditions in the ring," says the New Jersey Boxing Commission.

That thinly veiled reference to AIDS is just one more example of the extraordinary responses to the fear of AIDS that crop up daily across the USA.

USA Today (September 28, 1987). Used by permission.

Coughing

"Pulmonary tuberculosis, combined with pulmonary AIDS, would be highly lethal because both the microbes would be coughed into the air, and both remain infectious for more than a week at room temperatures."

Dr. Seale, M.D., *AIDS: A Special Report* (Noebel/Cameron/Lutton), p. 155.

"Persons with AIDS who are coughing should cover their mouths with tissues or handkerchiefs."

AIDS: A Special Report (Noebel/Cameron/Lutton), p. 155.

Dental Drills

Your dentist may not be an AIDS carrier, but his drill could be! Dr. Balbir Bagga, professor of dentistry at the University of Illinois, declared that most dentists use old hand-held drills which hold germ-laden water from one patient's mouth and deposit it into the mouth of the next patient! Dr. Bagga said, "This is definitely a danger with AIDS. Viruses like AIDS grow in the machine and then are transmitted from one patient to the next."

Dr. Balbir Bagga, Professor of Dentistry, University of Illinois

Casual Contact

Ear Piercing

Once a critical mass of the population has been infected with the virus, by highly efficient means of transmission, then less efficient means inevitably become more common. These include blood transfusions, transmission from mother to newborn babe, biologically normal sexual intercourse, needle-stick to nursing staff, chance contact of blood, saliva or sputum with sores or abrasions at home, at work, and at play. And, biting insects and flies, acupuncture, tatooing, ear-piercing, blood brother rituals, and routine dental procedures.

Dr. John Seale, *AIDS: A Special Report: Health and Human Services Committee* (Noebel/Lutton/Cameron, September 29, 1986).

Eyes Invaded Via Mucous Membrane

If a health care worker has a parenteral (for example, needle stick or cut) or mucous membrane (for example, splash to the eye or mouth) exposure to blood or other body fluids, the source patient should be assessed clinically and epidemiologically to determine the likelihood of HTLV-III/LAV infection. If the assessment suggests that infection may exist, the patient would be informed of the incident and requested to consent to serologic testing for evidence of HTLV-III/LAV infection.

JAMA-(Journal of the American Medical Association) Morbidity and Mortality Weekly Report: "Summary: Recommendation for Preventing Transmission of Infection With HTLV-III/LAV in the Workplace" (1985) Vol. 34, No. 45.

Food Handlers

Dr. Selma Dritz of the San Francisco Department of Health wrote in the *Western Journal of Medicine* saying, "Special precautions are required to protect the public from [carriers] who work as food handlers, bartenders, atten-

Dr. Dritz, *Western Journal of Medicine.*

dants in medical-care facilities, and as teachers and aids in day-care facilities for infants and young children. Common sense suggests that sexually active gays have no business in any of these occupations.

Dr. Selma Dritz, *Western Journal of Medicine*: (San Francisco Health Department).

Food Handlers

Because the virus is found in numerous body fluids, it would be reasonable and prudent to exclude carriers of the virus from occupations which involve direct touch contact with the public, or which involve food handling. No person carrying HTLV-III/LAV virus should be working in a profession which requires a health department license, or working in a facility which is subject to sanitary inspection. This would include beauticians, physicians, dentists, dental technicians, nurses and other health professionals, as well as food-service workers. These persons could be screened in a manner similar to the present military screening process. By utilizing objective tests for the actual virus, one would place the situation in the proper public-health context.

John Grauerholz, M.D., *EIR, Executive Intelligence Review*: "Why the AIDS Pandemic Requires a National Public Health Mobilization" (September 27, 1985), Vol. 12 No. 38.

Food Handlers

Dr. Sidney Finegold, president of the Infectious Disease Society of America [said], "It would seem prudent to ask that AIDS patients not engage in food preparation or handling for others." Every food handler should be tested for various communicable diseases.

Dr. Sidney Finegold, President of the Infectious Disease Society of America

Casual Contact

Food Handlers

No AIDS carrier should be permitted to work at any school, hospital, clinic, nursing home, or restaurant. It seems reasonable, therefore, that AIDS victims should not work as dental or medical technicians and should probably not be employed as food handlers. Would YOU want a dentist with AIDS working in your mouth, or how about a surgeon performing surgery on you? When you eat your next meal in a restaurant, think about the chef preparing your meal with a small cut on his hand. And your chef has AIDS!

Dr. Richard Restak, *Washington Post* (September 8, 1985).

Food Handlers
AIDS No Bar for U.S. Meat Inspectors

WASHINGTON — Federal meat and poultry inspectors who get AIDS can remain on the job as long as their work is acceptable and they don't come down with another contagious disease, the Agriculture Department says.

"If all they had was AIDS, they would not be removed from the plant situation just because they had the disease ... unless it was determined they couldn't do their job," Karen Stuck, a spokeswoman for the department's Food Safety and Inspection Service, said.

Stuck said it has been the agency's policy to remove inspectors from duties in cases of contagious disease. Only if an inspector developed a contagious disease in addition to AIDS would the worker be ordered off the job, the agency said. *(What a joke. — JVI)*

Last month, a senior official of the department's inspection agency, Lester Crawford, said the department had no reason to believe AIDS can be transmitted through food, but meat packing industry officials had expressed fear that

Kendall, *Detroit News* (October 29, 1987).

the disease could be passed through blood from knife cuts and other injuries common among plant workers.

(Notice the danger — blood on the meat created from cuts. How about salads? — JVI)

Don Kendall, *Detroit News* (Associated Press, October 29, 1987).

Football Players
New AIDS Plans Include Education,
New Training Rules

Concern among football players rests primarily with the possibility of transmitting the fatal disease from one player with an open wound to another who also has an open wound.

Athletic teams are different from other workers because they live in such close proximity, using the same shower and training facilities.

"It's a very serious question," quarterback Eric Hipple said. "It's a bloody game. You're mixing blood with a lot of people.

"That's the concern of the players: The protection against disease."

Hipple is in favor of testing for AIDS, which is not legal.

"No player should be attacked for wanting to have testing," Hipple said. "It's not an attack against a certain lifestyle. When you hear people say they want it (testing), I think they're not saying they want the homosexuals out. They're not trying to pinpoint anybody, and they're not trying to find out who a gay player might be.

"Football is a bloody game. You bleed. There are times when that blood is mixed with other players' in contact. That's a legitimate beef by the players."

The Detroit News (July 30, 1987).

Casual Contact

Funeral Directors

When funeral directors are called to take charge of remains, they should definitely be told the cause of death. There are precautionary measures that we take when handling a communicable diseased body. If a worker's hand is accidentally punctured while handling a body, his safety could be jeopardized.

Thomas Delehanty, Funeral Director, Loves Park, Illinois.

Jewish Ruling on AIDS Bodies

Jewish burial societies have been told that neither religious laws nor tradition requires them to wash bodies of AIDS victims.

The ruling was made last month and disclosed yesterday.

Rabbinical experts at Yeshiva University said the ruling "probably" freed burial societies from two other forms of intimate contact with the dead — trimming of finger and toe nails and combing or cutting of hair.

The ruling by rabbinical experts in Jewish law came at the request of a rabbi who said members of some burial societies were afraid that contact with AIDS victims might infect them.

"It is a question that every Jewish community is now addressing," said Rabbi Yitzchak Rosenbaum, professor of Jewish law at Yeshiva University, the leading center for Orthodox education in the United States.

Charles W. Bell, *Daily News* (July 10, 1987).

Insects
Time Will Tell

Specimens of numerous insects [mosquitos, cockroaches, tsetse flies, etc.] from central Africa have been found to contain the AIDS virus, according to French scientists, who

New York Times (August 27, 1986).

stressed that, despite the discovery, transmission of AIDS to humans by insects was extremely unlikely.

The New York Times (August 27, 1986), p.A-10

Kissing Note:
Deep Kissing Refers to French Kissing

According to Dr. Dean Echenberg of the San Francisco Health Department, the AIDS virus has been found in saliva. He feels that the exchange of saliva (as occurs in deep, passionate kissing) is putting an individual at grave risk ...

Dr. Dean Echenberg, San Francisco Department of Health

Broken Skin

Open-mouth kissing where exchange of saliva occurs, is regarded as somewhat dangerous, as is kissing anywhere the skin has been broken.

Cheek kissing is safe. At this time, I can't be any more definite about this.

Dr. Paul Donohue, *Detroit News*: "Your Health."

Intimacy

In reply to the question, "Is kissing safe?" Dr. James Slaff, of the National Institutes of Health replied, "No." He went on to say, "Given the available evidence, intimate kissing should be considered a risky activity by infected and uninfected individuals alike."

Dr. James Slaff, National Institutes of Health

There is a risk of infecting others by ... exposure of others to saliva through oral-generated contact of intimate kissing.

Noebel/Lutton/Cameron, *ISIS Newsletter*: "Special Report: AIDS" (July/August 1985), Centers for Disease Control, January 11, 1985, MMWR.

Casual Contact

French Kissing

Is kissing safe? No. Current United States Food and Drug Administration and World Health Organization guidelines to individuals who have had a positive blood test showing antibodies to the AIDS virus specifically recommend that infected individuals refrain from intimate or "French" kissing.

United States Food and Drug Administration, World Health Organization

According to current draft federal recommendations (MMWR, 1985; 34: p. 1-5):

Each person with a positive test would have to be told (in gentle, carefully worded phrases) that they cannot engage in sexual intercourse, kiss someone, or seek medical or dental care without possibly exposing their partner or health care provider to this possible deadly virus.

Joel L. Nitzkin, M.D./Mark J. Merkens, M.D., *JAMA-(Journal of the American Medical Association)* (June 21, 1985), Vol. 253 No. 23.

Altering Lifestyle Can Avert AIDS — Hugging Not a Problem

Can people get AIDS by kissing and hugging someone who carries the virus?

"Dry" kissing is considered safe. Deep, "wet" kissing is not recommended because low levels of virus have been found in saliva of infected people. Hugging is not a problem.

Mary McGath, *World Herald* Medical Writer (October 25, 1987).

AIDS Transmitted to Elderly Wife Via Kissing

Jerome Groopman and others at the National Institutes of Health discovered the AIDS virus in the saliva of AIDS carriers. They concluded, "The recovery of HTLV/III from saliva suggests that direct contact with this body fluid

Drs. Groopman, Slaff, Salahuddin

should be avoided since saliva ... could facilitate horizontal (person-to-person) transmission."

And Dr. James Slaff of the National Institutes of Health has stated, "Because the AIDS virus has been cultured from the saliva of infected individuals, the FDA currently recommends that infected individuals refrain from 'French' kissing. This is a reasonable precaution. Dr. Zaki Salahuddin has provided an example in which intimate kissing was the only possible vector of transmission: an elderly infected woman whose only exposure was kissing her AIDS husband, an impotent transfusion recipient."

Drs. Groopman, Slaff, & Salahuddin, National Institutes of Health

Illinois Pathologists: Pathologists Must Guard Against AIDS

Your recent editorial about reporting AIDS deaths provided inaccurate information by referring only to "undertakers and forensic pathologists" as using special precautions when handling bodies of AIDS victims. In fact, many pathologists, not only those physicians who have specialized in forensic pathology, often perform autopsies on persons who have died of AIDS and other contagious diseases. *Use of special safety procedures is the routine in all autopsy procedures when a diagnosis is uncertain.* As the ultimate medical audit, the autopsy benefits the living and future generations.

William Kuehn, *Letterline* (Skokie, Illinois).

Saliva

Can the virus be transmitted by saliva? Under some circumstances we believe this may occur with intimate contact, ...

Robert C. Gallo, M.D./Flossie Wong-Staal, Ph.D., *Annals of Internal Medicine*: "A Human T-Lymphotropic Retrovirus (HTLV-III) as the Cause of the Acquired Immunodeficiency Syndrome" (1985), Vol. 103, p. 684.

Casual Contact

Saliva

The human immunodeficiency virus [AIDS] can be transmitted through exposure to blood and possibly through contact with other bodily fluids, such as saliva. Thus, infection with HIV is a potential hazard for health care and laboratory workers ...

Individual case reports of AIDS among health care workers without known risk factors have occurred ...

J. M. Mann, M.D., MPH/H. Francis, M.D./T. C. Quinn, M.D./K. Bila, M.D./P. K. Asila, M.D., MPH/N. Bosenge, M.D./N. Nzilambi, M.D./L. Jansegers, M.D./P. Pilot, M.D./K. Ruti, M.D./J. W. Curran, M.D, MPH, *JAMA-(Journal of American Medical Association):* "HIV Seroprevalence Among Hospital Workers in Kinshasha, Zaire" (December 12, 1986), Vol. 256 No. 22.

Saliva

Dr. William Hazeltine [sic] stated, "Anyone who tells you categorically that AIDS is not contracted by saliva is not telling you the truth. AIDS may, in fact, be transmissible by tears, saliva, body fluids, and mosquito bites."

Alan M. Dershowitz, *The New York Times*: "Emphasize Scientific Information" (March 18, 1986).

Skin

Three hospital workers developed AIDS virus infections after their skin was exposed briefly to the blood of patients infected with the deadly disease, [said] researchers at the U.S. Centers for Disease Control.

The new cases, involving three women from separate parts of the country, marked the first documented cases of AIDS infections among health workers in which spread of the virus did not involve direct injection of infected blood

News Record (May 20, 1987).

into the body or prolonged exposure to direct body fluids of an infected patient.

News Record: "Hospital Workers Develop AIDS" (Associated Press, May 20, 1987).

Skin
3 Get AIDS in New Way

ATLANTA (AP) — Three hospital workers whose skin came in brief contact with the blood of patients infected with the AIDS virus developed the potentially deadly infection themselves, according to reports published today.

The new cases, involving women in different parts of the country, mark the first documented cases involving health-care workers in which spread of the virus did not involve direct injection of infected blood into the body or prolonged exposure to an AIDS patient's body fluids, the reports said.

The Centers for Disease Control said hospital workers should follow strict precautions but not be alarmed and stressed there was still no evidence that acquired immune deficiency syndrome can be transmitted through casual contact.

The new cases documented by the CDC were reported by the *Atlanta Constitution*, the *New York Times*, and the *Washington Post*.

One of the cases involved a worker who also had blood spattered into her mouth when she was drawing blood from an infected patient, he said.

"The take-home message here is that it emphasizes that health-care workers coming into contact with blood should follow certain precautions," he said.

The CDC has previously advocated such precautions, including wearing gloves, masks, gowns and eye protection, in handling AIDS patients.

Tulsa Tribune

Casual Contact

Curran said each of the women had chapped hands, dermatitis or breaks in the skin through which the AIDS virus might have passed.

The woman who was splattered in the mouth might have become infected when the virus passed across the mucous membrane in her mouth *or possibly through an inflamed area on her face, he said.*

The federal agency summoned more than 20 state public health officials, hospital infection control experts, and American Hospital Association officials to Atlanta last week to discuss the three cases, Curran said.

Details of the cases are to [be] published Thursday in the CDC's *Morbidity and Mortality Weekly Report.*

In four previously reported cases, health care workers apparently were infected with the virus after accidentally sticking themselves with hypodermic needles that had been used to treat AIDS patients. *Two other health care workers who became infected were women who cared for AIDS-infected patients and were constantly exposed to the patients' blood, urine, and other bodily fluids.*

The Tulsa Tribune, (Tulsa, Oklahoma).

Sperm
Death Sentence of AIDS

Our study, with its well-defined source and timing of virus contact, has some unique aspects with respect to the epidemiology of HTLV-III infection in women. It indicates that the virus can be transmitted by semen (sperm) implanted in the vagina without bodily contact.

G. J. Stewart/J.P.P. Tyler/ A. L. Cunningham/J. A. Barr/ G. L. Driscoll/ J. Gold/B. J. Lamont, *Lancet:* "Transmission of Human T-Cell Lymphotropic Virus Type III (HTLV-III) by Artificial Insemination Donor" (September 14, 1985).

Artificial Insemination

There have been four babies in Australia born with AIDS because the sperm donor had AIDS. Artificial insemination is not a safe alternative.

Cory SerVaas, M.D., *The Saturday Evening Post*: "Help Prevent the Spread of AIDS" (January/February 1986).

Promiscuity, the resulting exposure, and immune responses to infectious agents and sperm are proposed to be the initiating and sustaining factors of AIDS.

J. Sonnabend, M.B., MRCP/S. Witkin, Ph.D./D. Purtilo, M.D., *JAMA-(Journal of the American Medical Association): AIDS: From the Beginning*: "Acquired Immunodeficiency Syndrome, Opportunistic Infections, and Malignancies in Male Homosexuals"

Tears

... I can't guarantee that the virus could not be spread through contact with tears. Certainly, *I wouldn't like to have tears with virus in it rubbed into an open wound on my arm ...*

Malcolm Martin, M.D., Chief, Laboratory of Molecular Microbiology, in the Infectious Diseases Institute.

Eye Care Professionals

Although the level of HIV in tears is low and there has been no documented instance, HIV transmission is theoretically possible. Therefore, eye care professionals are advised to take appropriate precautions, including wearing gloves when sterilizing or disinfecting instruments, and disinfecting contact lenses.

Federal Drug Administration (October 1985).

Teeth: Biting

A prison inmate who bit two guards after testing positive for AIDS was found guilty Wednesday of two counts of assault with a deadly and dangerous weapon — his mouth

Star Tribune (June 25, 1987).

and teeth.

Moore was accused of biting guards Timothy Voight and Ronald McCullough at the Federal Medical Center in Rochester, Minnesota, in January.

During the trial, Assistant U.S. Attorney Jon Hopeman said Moore told a nurse after the incident that he wanted the guards to die and hoped they would get AIDS from the wounds.

Star Tribune: "Inmate With AIDS Who Bit Guards Convicted by Jury" (Associated Press, June 25, 1987).

Summary
An Opposing View

Don Boys — Indianapolis House of Representatives — Fear Is Well-founded; So Is Discrimination

INDIANAPOLIS — I plead guilty to discrimination. When I bought an Olds instead of a Ford, I proved my guilt. When I married a blonde instead of a fiery redhed, I discriminated. I discriminate daily. And I believe it is my right and duty to do so!

I choose to associate with decent, clean-living, clear-thinking people — people who have a measure of civility that has been distilled over the centuries. I will not knowingly surround myself, personally or professionally, with fornicators, drunks, thieves, rapists, sodomites, or people with a corrupt vocabulary.

Dr. Richard Restak said, "It seems reasonable ... that AIDS victims should not ... work as dental or medical technicians, and should probably not be employed as food handlers."

Would you want a surgeon with AIDS operating on you?

Boys, *USA Today* (December 3, 1986).

Casual Contact

Would you want the chef at your favorite restaurant, an AIDS carrier, preparing your meal with a cut on his hand? The AIDS virus has been found in all the bodily fluids. Harvard pathologist William Haseltine said, "Nobody can give you an absolute guarantee that one out of 100,000 times someone isn't going to transmit it on a drinking glass or through sweat. All we can say, and all we should say, is that so far, to our knowledge, it hasn't happened."

We who are skeptical about the shallow assurances from political physicians as to casual contact with AIDS carriers are accused of being producers of panic. We are made to appear irresponsible by the irresponsible ones! We are made to appear as bigots by the bigots! It's the old game of slander your opponent when you can't or won't answer his charges.

Non-thinking liberals tell us it is wrong to be critical of sodomites, but not wrong to be critical of those who are critical of sodomites! Such people have rexophobia — an inordinate, irrational fear of moral normalcy. It seems many liberals have a knee-jerk reaction — left one, of course — to anything patriotic, decent, normal, and especially Christian.

Don Boys, Indianapolis House of Representatives, *USA Today* (December 3, 1986). Used by permission.

Condoms

The Surgeon General is now seen daily on TV urging people to use condoms and practice "safe sex." He is not seen on TV, however, alerting the American Public to the fact that the condom is not safe. He does not say that, depending on the type of sexual activity, the condom can fail 3 or 5 out of 10 times — allowing this disease to continue its insidious spread.

Judie Brown, American Life League, Inc.

The teaching of use of condoms has been widely argued. It is abused to promote the virtues of an appliance that even the homosexual community rejects as useless. *The Gay Advocate* condemns the condom as a safeguard.

Education Reporter: "Legislation Update" (April 1987), No. 15.

Dr. James Goedert said, "Condoms probably reduce the risk of catching AIDS, but they are no guarantee ..."

News Record: "Report Urges AIDS Testing of All Sexually Active Adults" (Associated Press, May 27, 1987).

Dr. John Seale told a Baltimore audience, "Relying upon condoms [to stop AIDS] is the equivalent of running into enemy lines wearing a tin hat and getting shot in the chest. You may think you're 'protected,' but you die anyway."

Seale said that promoting condom use as a way of stopping AIDS is "more likely to accelerate the spread of the virus ... than to stop it." Seale believes the answer is not in condoms but common sense. He urged activists in Virginia to work to protect the rights of the uninfected and urged universal AIDS testing!

Dr. John Seale, Health and Human Services Committee

The idea of using condoms ... is a half measure. It's like putting a band-aid over a hemorrhage. It simply isn't going to contain the problem.

Dr. Vernon A. Mark, Associate Professor of Surgery, Harvard Medical School, Interview with Dr. Ed Rowe, President, New National AIDS Prevention Institute

The simple fact is that the overwhelming means by which AIDS is transmitted are through blood exchanges (transfusion, shared needles, etc.) and anal intercourse (condoms help, but offer no guarantee of safety). With greatly improved techniques for screening donated blood, the two groups remaining greatly at risk are homosexual men and intravenous drug abusers.

William Raspberry, *The Detroit News* (November 1, 1987).

Recent studies reported in the press have indicated that natural membrane condoms are not able to contain — and, therefore, are unable to protect against infection from — the HIV virus. Therefore, FDA allows only latex condoms to be labeled for the prevention of STD's including AIDS.

Federal Drug Administration

In a study found in the Feb. 6, 1987 *Journal of the American Medical Association*, University of Miami School of Medicine Doctors Fischl, Dickinson, et.al., found that of the ten couples who used "barrier contraceptives" one couple developed the AIDS virus for a ten percent transmission ratio. Since the report, however, it has been confirmed by Dr. Gordon M. Dickinson that two more couples have transmitted the AIDS virus for a thirty percent transmission rate. A British medical journal, *The Lancet*, for December 21/28, 1985, found that condoms split during "anal inter-

JAMA (February 6, 1987).

Condoms

course" up to fifty percent of the time. States *Lancet*, "This is an important observation in the light of recommendations that condoms be used by homosexual men during anal intercourse." Condoms may delay passage of the AIDS virus, but they will not prevent the spread of the lethal disease. *The truth is simple: there is no "safe sex" with anyone infected with AIDS.*

Journal of the American Medical Association (February 6, 1987).

Some experts, such as Dr. Michael Rosenberg of the American Social Health Association, a group that tracks sexually transmitted diseases, estimate that condoms may reduce the chances of getting AIDS by about half. That's about the protection they afford for other sexually transmitted diseases. But no one has good numbers. Since condoms burst and others are removed too soon or otherwise used incorrectly, says Rosenberg, we still need to know: Do condom users use condoms all the time? If so, why do they fail? Is it product failure, or noncompliance?

Projects to help find answers are under way. One will include lab tests of 35 condom brands and spermicides, plus clinical trials to see how well they work against AIDS in homosexuals and heterosexuals. Anecdotal reports suggest that anal sex, a common practice among gays and a small proportion of heterosexuals, damages condoms. Results of the trials won't be available for at least six months.

U.S. News & World Report (October 19, 1987).

We have no reliable figures on the safety of condoms for preventing AIDS. Preliminary studies demonstrate that they delay infection but do not prevent it ... "Safe sex" practices centering around the use of condoms are not as safe as the public has been led to believe. While in most labo-

Dr. Crenshaw (February 10, 1987).

ratory experiments they do not pass sperm, herpes or the AIDS virus, in practice, they have a 10 percent failure rate for pregnancy (per woman per year). A woman is able to get pregnant only three to five days a month. She is susceptible to AIDS 365 days a year. Sperm are 500 times larger than a virus. Condoms leak and condoms break. Often overlooked is the fact that sexual arousal is much like alcohol intoxication. The first thing to go is your judgment. Taking these factors into consideration, common sense suggests that the failure rate for the AIDS virus would be much higher than 10 percent.

Dr. Theresa L. Crenshaw, House Subcommittee on Health (February 10, 1987).

Dr. Margaret Fischal, an American Medical Associate: "Condoms appeared to decrease the incidence of transmission but did not decrease it to zero level. The only guarantee was abstinence."

News Record: "Abstinence Only Guarantee Against Disease," (Associated Press, February 11, 1987).

We can do something about the problem of AIDS. As a people we can stop this if we have the will to do it and this does not mean by using ... condoms. It means changing our sexual behavior and if we do that, we have the ability to stop this dreaded potential plague in its tracks.

Dr. Vernon A. Mark, Associate Professor of Surgery, Harvard Medical School, Interview with Dr. Ed Rowe, President, New AIDS Prevention Institute.

You've got to remember that if, even in marriage, if one partner is promiscuous, their marriage partner is not only having sex with them, that person, but also having sex with every individual that person has ever had sex with so that

Drs. Mark, Rowe (March 1987).

Condoms

over a period of how many sexual partners that the promiscuous one may have sex with, they're putting their own marriage partner at tremendous risk by doing this.

Dr. Vernon A. Mark, Associate Professor of Surgery, Harvard Medical School, Interview with Dr. Ed Rowe, President, New National AIDS Prevention Institute (March 1987).

If you are a parent concerned about sexually promiscuous programming on evening television, brace yourself — some new commercials may be even worse than the shows themselves. The commercials advertise condoms and are now being shown on a number of local television stations across the country.

What is objectionable about these TV commercials is not so much what they are promoting, but how they are promoting it. The ads tout condoms as the answer to public concern over the spread of AIDS (Acquired Immune Deficiency Syndrome). They suggest that, with condoms, one can have it all — a sexually promiscuous lifestyle and protection from sexually transmitted diseases. For example, one ad features a young, curly-haired girl who says, "I'll do a lot for love. But I'm not ready to die for it."

What is missing from these ads is any notion that sexual relations are somehow associated with marriage. Indeed, one soon gets the impression from these commercials that condoms are no longer taboo — but monogamous, heterosexual relations are!

That message troubles me because I am concerned about our nation's youth and the kind of values we pass on to them. It troubles me because the impression is given that a medical seal of approval is yours against AIDS if you will just use the condoms. And it troubles me because I believe the best way to thwart the spread of AIDS is to encourage

Regeir, Family Research Council.

people to abstain from sexual intercourse outside of marriage. While abstinence may not be appealing to some segments of our society, I am confident that it, like honesty, is the best policy.

Gerald P. Regier, President, Family Research Council of America, Inc.

25-40 Million With V.D.

If you haven't heard yet, condom ads are "on the air."

The explanation is something like this: "AIDS IS A deadly disease that has already killed 18,285 people — in the United States alone! Another 31,834 have contracted the disease and most of these will be dead in two years or so. And beyond these two devastating figures, another one to two million Americans carry the virus and many, most, or all will eventually contract the disease and die as well.

"So, America needs to protect itself from AIDS. In other words, Americans need 'safe sex.' And the best way to have 'safe sex' is to use condoms. And the best way to get the American public to use this 1865 invention is to put condom ads on television."

There you have it.

Are you finished laughing? Have you started crying?

Let's put this startling suggestion in proper perspective.

AMERICA is not just now having to combat a destructive sexually transmitted disease.

At this very moment, millions upon millions of Americans suffer from any one or more of 25 sexually transmitted diseases.

In 1985 alone, there were 27,143 newly reported cases of syphilis, 910,895 cases of gonorrhea, 1 million cases of genital warts, 1 million cases of urethritis, 1.2 million cases of mucopurulent cervi citis, and 4 million cases of chlamydia.

And that's not all.

Mawyer, *Liberty Report.*

Condoms

There are, perhaps, between 5 to 10 million people with genital herpes. And some estimate that the total number of people suffering from genital warts is between 25 to 40 million!

The consequences of these sexually transmitted diseases range from itching, pain, and embarrassment, to brain damage, cancer, and death.

The condom has been around for well over a century.

WHO HASN'T heard, who doesn't know that condoms will reduce the risk of sexually transmitted diseases?

Are we really to believe that 25 years after the beginning of the sexual revolution, 25 years after the world's largest onslaught of humiliation and death through sexually transmitted diseases that there are still people copulating who don't know about condoms?

Of course not.

So why put them on television?

This has got to be the medical profession's most embarrassing answer to a disease since the introduction of bloodletting as a medical cure-all.

There are only two answers to sexually transmitted diseases: abstinence and monogamous relationships.

That's all.

But society — which has grown fond of the saying, "If it feels good, do it" — is not about to stop having casual sex.

Martin Mawyer, *Liberty Report*.

AIDS
New Definition of Aids Disease
Sends Case Count Higher

Many AIDS patients have developed severe dementia including memory loss, slurred speech and psychoses. Doctors had attributed these symptoms to the patients' general decline until 1985, when Dr. Martin S. Hirsch, a virologist at the Massachusetts General Hospital, suggested the virus might be invading and destroying nerve cells.

"I expect there will be a jump over the course of a month or two," said Dr. Tim Dondero, chief of the surveillance and evaluation branch for the CDC's AIDS program.

"We know that a number of states have a backlog of cases initially picked up and labeled 'suspect' cases or 'AIDS-like disease,' that will not qualify as AIDS under the new definition. How long it takes to report them, we don't know."

Kathleen Bohland, *Detroit News* (November 2, 1987).

Forgetfulness

Every time he forgets a phone number or leaves a pot on the stove these days, Aladar Marberger worries that he may be losing his mind. Recently, the 40-year-old New York art dealer started to tell some friends about his favorite hotel in Venice, the Cipriani, but stopped in midsentence, unable to recall its name. Oh, ... he thought. It's happening. And while he tells the story lightheartedly, Marberger — who 18 months ago was diagnosed with Kaposi's sarcoma, the cancer that is a hallmark of acquired immune deficiency syndrome — can't laugh off the reality: AIDS does not limit itself to the destruction of its victim's bodies. It often consumes their minds as well.

It's a part of the AIDS epidemic that the public knows

U.S. News & World Report (September 7, 1987).

Dementia

little about, and patients themselves prefer not to dwell on. Scientists call it AIDS-related dementia, and they are just beginning to decipher how the syndrome works. For their own part, AIDS patients call it the most terrifying thing they can imagine: The crumbling of humanity — often in the very prime of life — as the AIDS virus assaults the central nervous system, attacking the victim's ability to think, feel, talk, and move. "I've had a glorious life, and I'm not the least bit frightened of death," says Marberger. "But the thought of losing one's mind — well, it frightens the _____ out of me."

No one knows exactly how widespread AIDS dementia is, but the numbers are higher than researchers once thought. Studies of the brains of AIDS patients after their death indicate that 50 percent had sustained central-nervous-system damage that can be traced directly to the virus associated with AIDS, and an additional 25 percent had nervous-system damage due to infections, cancer, or stroke. One researcher, Dr. Richard Price of Memorial Sloan-Kettering Cancer Center, says it's possible that nearly two-thirds of the 15,000 AIDS patients in the United States will show symptoms of dementia before they die. And it's not just adults. In a study of 68 children with AIDS, pediatric neurologist Anita Belman of the State University of New York found that 61 had nervous-system problems such as spasticity or the inability to learn to speak ....

Dr. Richard Price, Dr. Anita Belman, *U.S. News & World Report*: "AIDS: Attacking the Brain" (Copyright, September 7, 1987, *U.S. News & World Report*). Used by permission.

Memory Loss

Many adult AIDS patients eventually develop the encephalopathy which characteristically begins with impaired concentration and mild memory loss and pro-

"HTLV-III Infection in Brains of Children and Adults With AIDS Encephalopathy."

gresses to severe global cognitive impairment ...

In children with AIDS, a similar constellation of neurologic abnormalities occurs.

G. M. Shaw/M. E. Harper/B. H. Hahn/L. G. Epstein/D. C. Gajdusek/ R. W. Price/B. A. Navia/C. K. Petito/C. J. O'Hara/J. E. Groopman Eun-Sook Cho/J. M. Oleske/F. Wond-Staal/R. C. Gallo, "HTLV-III Infection in Brains of Children and Adults With AIDS Encephalopathy."

Brain Atrophy

The ability of the AIDS virus to infect the central nervous system may account for the psychosis and brain atrophy that is common in patients.

Jeffrey Laurence, Ph.D., *Scientific American*: "The Immune System in AIDS" (December 1985).

Dementia — Disorientation and Death

... The advanced and terminal stages of the disease are especially frightening and painful ... a recent report has linked this dementia with the presence of human T-lymphotropic virus type III (HTLV-III) in the brain; ... this finding has raised questions about the possible similarities between HTLV-III and visna virus, which causes chronic degenerative neurologic disease in sheep.

The early clinical picture of this encephalopathy resembles depression and is often indistinguishable without neuropsychologic testing. *Usual initial symptoms are forgetfulness and poor concentration.* Psychomotor retardation, decreased alertness, apathy, withdrawal, diminished interest in work, and loss of libido develop soon after. Over several months, frank confusion, disorientation, seizures, mutism, profound dementia, coma, and death ensue.

J. C. Holland, M.D./S. Tross, Ph.D., *Annals of Internal Medicine*: "The Psychosocial and Neuropsychiatric Sequelae of the Acquired Immunodeficiency Syndrome and Related Disorders" (1985), Vol. 103.

Dementia

The syndrome of dementia in patients with AIDS due to this infection is becoming relatively well defined.

D. Armstrong, M.D./J.W.M. Gold, M.D./J. Dryjanski, M.D./E. Whimbey, M.D./B. Plosky, M.D./C. Hawkins, M.D./A. E. Brown, M.D./E. Bernard, B.A./T. E. Kiehn, Ph. D., *Annals of Internal Medicine*: "Treatment of Infections in Patients With the Acquired Immunodeficiency Syndrome" (1985), Vol. 103.

Dr. Koop has been a featured guest on our national telecast. While I greatly admire the man, I have been perplexed by some of his recent statements. His surgeon general's report on page six floored me. It is the joke of the century. I quote:

"You may have wondered why your dentist wears gloves and perhaps a mask when treating you. This does not mean that he has AIDS or that he thinks you do. He is protecting you and himself from hepatitis, common colds, or flu."

Come now, Dr. Koop. These viruses have been around for years. Why did dentists wait until now to protect themselves? Let's allow the public to judge this statement on the basis of expert testimony.

"When patients see the family dentist wearing gloves, mask and glasses, they should be reassured, not threatened."

Edward Barrett, president of the Academy of General Dentistry, on a new survey of dentists indicating that nearly all wear gloves and masks when treating patients they suspect of carrying the AIDS virus and that 78 percent now wear gloves when treating all patients.

Edward Barrett, *U.S. News & World Report* (December 21, 1987).

Masks and Gloves

The Centers of Disease Control on November 15, 1985, and April 11, 1986, issued recommendations for preventing transmission of AIDS between dentists and patients. These recommendations, including the wearing of masks and gloves, have been adopted by the nation's dentists.

Phoebe Courtney, *The Independent American*: "Can AIDS Threaten You?" (February 1987), No. 217.

An Infected Dentist

Dental health workers are in professional contact with a large number of patients, most of whom appear to be healthy. However, because a large proportion of persons infected with HIV do not show signs of infection, it is urgent that dental health workers take measures to protect themselves as well as their patients from HIV transmission. A recent report at the International Conference on AIDS, of a dentist who frequently practiced without gloves and who apparently contracted HIV from a patient, emphasizes the importance of following infection control procedures.

CDC has published infection control recommendations for dental health workers that may serve to prevent transmission of HIV as well as other microorganisms. Dentists and others in dentistry are urged to refer to the complete recommendations referenced at the end of this article. Summarized, they include:

Gloves

Gloves must always be worn when touching blood, saliva, or mucous membranes; when touching blood-soiled items, body fluids, or secretions, as well as surfaces contaminated with them; and when examining all oral lesions.

All work must be completed on one patient, where possible, and the gloves removed and the hands washed and regloved before performing procedures on another patient.

Repeated use of a single pair of gloves is not recommended, since such use is likely to produce defects in the glove material that will diminish its value as an effective barrier.

FDA Drug Bulletin (September 1987).

Hands must be washed between patients (following removal of gloves), after touching inanimate objects likely to be contaminated by blood or saliva from other patients, and before leaving the operatory. During use, gloves may become perforated, whether or not the operator is aware of it. This allows viral contamination as well as allowing bacteria to enter and multiply beneath the glove material. For many routine dental procedures, hand washing with plain soap appears to be adequate. For surgical procedures, an antimicrobial scrub should be used.

Protective Masks and Gowns

Surgical masks and protective eyewear or chin-length plastic face shields must be worn when splashing or spattering of blood or other body fluids is likely, as is common in dentistry.

Reusable or disposable gowns, lab coats, or uniforms must be worn when clothing is likely to be soiled with blood or other body fluids. If reusable gowns are worn, they may be washed, using a normal laundry cycle. Gowns should be changed at least daily or when visibly soiled with blood.

Instruments and Surfaces

Impervious-backed paper, aluminum foil, or clear plastic wrap may be used to cover surfaces that may be contaminated by blood or saliva and that are difficult or impossible to clean and disinfect. These coverings should be removed (while gloved), discarded, and then replaced (after ungloving) with clean material between patients.

Instruments that penetrate soft tissue and/or bone

FDA Drug Bulletin (September 1987).

Dentists

should be sterilized after each use. Instruments that are not intended to penetrate oral soft tissue or bone but that may come into contact with oral tissue should also be sterilized after each use if possible; however, if sterilization is not feasible, the latter instruments should receive high-level disinfection.

Metal and heat-stable dental instruments should be routinely sterilized between uses by autoclaving, dry heat, or chemical vapor.

Routine sterilization of handpieces (drills) between patients is desirable. In the case of handpieces that cannot be sterilized, other complete cleaning and disinfection procedures should be followed. The same is true of ultrasonic scalers and air/water syringes.

Because water retraction valves within the dental units may aspirate infective materials back into the handpiece and water line, these valves should be replaced with a non-aspirating method of coolant water containment.

FDA Drug Bulletin (September 1987).

Disinformation and Distortion

Marla Minnicino opened her article in the *New Federalist* by quoting British AIDS expert, Dr. John Seale: "The scientific basis of 'safe sex' educating now being promoted by governments to children all over the world is based upon carefully presented disinformation and distortion of the truth emanating from internationally renowned scientists and public health doctors."

But Dr. Seale got more specific. He accused scientists of betraying a "sacred trust." He then named seven international officials whom he feels are jeopardizing the public welfare and leading to many deaths! He lists Dr. Everett Koop, Surgeon General of the U.S., as number one!

Marla Minnicino, *New Federalist*

Centers for Disease Control Discredited

UNITED NATIONS, Nov. 20 (NSIPS) — In an extraordinary self-confessional press conference yesterday, Dr. Halfdan Mahler, the Danish director general of the World Health Organization (WHO), called AIDS "a health disaster of pandemic proportions" and predicted that conservatively there would be 100 million infected with the disease within five years.

Heretofore the WHO has been leading a global disinformation campaign to downplay the threat of AIDS, in coordination with the now-collapsing and discredited Centers for Disease Control (CDC) in the United States.

Last year, at a press conference in Zambia, Dr. Mahler said that people should keep AIDS in perspective to other diseases and should not overplay its threat. At his UN press conference, however, Dr. Mahler admitted that he had not had "a feeling for what was brewing with regard to AIDS.

"I thought wait and see — maybe it is not as hot as some are making it appear," he said. "I definitely admit to a gross underestimate."

Warren J. Hamerman, Director, EIR Biological Holocaust Task Force

Disinformation and Distortion

CDC Cover-up Exposed

The collective malfeasance in the leadership of the CDC and their AIDS program was first publicly exposed 13 months ago in a 10-page documentary feature in the journal *Executive Intelligence Review* (EIR), titled "Why Is the Atlanta CDC Covering Up the AIDS Story?" (EIR, Vol. 12 No. 38, p. 52-61, September 27, 1985).

The policies which have brought the nation to the brink of an AIDS catastrophe were ordered from White House Chief of Staff Don Regan through CDC Director James Mason, for "budgetary reasons" (EIR: "Don Regan Charged With Cover-up on AIDS Spread," Vol. 13 No. 41, p. 20-29, October 17, 1986).

Now the National Academy of Sciences report has exposed the Pollyanna statements of the CDC as "politically" motivated distortions.

Projections of a Catastrophe

Among the summary of the new National Academy of Sciences report are the following points:

- There is a likely tenfold increase for AIDS cases over the next five years.
- Anyone who has antibodies to the virus must be assumed to be infected and probably capable of transmitting the virus.
- A person infected with HIV may not show any clinical symptoms for months or even years, but apparently never becomes free of the virus. This long, often unrecognized period of asymptomatic infection, during which an infected person can infect others, complicates control of the spread of the virus.

EIR (September 27, 1985).

- There have been 24,500 AIDS cases and an additional 50,000 to 125,000 ARC cases already counted.
- At least 25 to 50% of infected persons will progress to AIDS within 5 to 10 years of infection. The possibility that the percentage is higher cannot be ruled out.
- By the end of 1991, there will have been a cumulative total of more than 270,000 cases of AIDS in the U.S., with more than 74,000 of those occurring in 1991 alone.
- By the end of 1991 there will have been a cumulative total of more than 179,000 American AIDS deaths, with more than 54,000 of those in 1991 alone.
- Because the typical time between infection and development of clinical AIDS is four or more years, most of the persons who will develop AIDS between now and 1991 are already infected.
- Pediatric AIDS cases will increase almost tenfold in the next five years.
- There will be substantially more cases in the heterosexual population over the next 5 to 10 years.
- There are an estimated 10 million individuals infected worldwide; the developing sector will suffer the most from the disease.

The IOM-NAS Committee on a National Strategy for AIDS is coordinated by an 11-scientist steering committee co-chaired by Dr. David Baltimore and Dr. Sheldon M. Wolff. In addition to the steering committee, the report was prepared by 23 additional scientists, grouped into a "Research Panel" and a "Health Care and Public Health Panel."

Executive Intelligence Review (Centers for Disease Control, September 27, 1985).

Disinformation and Distortion

Medical Experts Criticize the Centers for Disease Control Because of the Following Reasons:

1. Covering up the true magnitude of the number of cases. First, CDC tried to restrict the definition of what should be called AIDS; now they are simply ignoring the results of studies, such as those of Drs. Engleman and Lifson, published last summer by the Stanford Medical School, which show that CDC is "massaging" the data downward, to report perhaps as few as one-tenth of the true number of cases.

2. Ignoring the existence of massive studies, some by CDC's own research teams, on the direct relationship between the rapid spread of AIDS, and conditions of economic collapse ...

3. Covering up the results of numerous studies *proving that it is medically unsound to allow children or teachers with AIDS into the school system* ...

4. Downplaying the efficacy of the blood screening test for identifying infected individuals. This is quite remarkable, since at the same time, CDC has been extolling the efficacy of the blood test for eliminating infected blood from the nation's blood supply.

5. Obfuscating the significance of factors of economic collapse, in accounting for the outbreak of AIDS in Belle Glade [Florida], among non-homosexuals and non-drug users.

6. Maintaining that AIDS is "only" a disease which can be transmitted to a restricted "risk" population, and not a general threat to society.

7. Medical and health professionals also generally agree that the CDC figures are vastly underestimated. Offi-

EIR (September 27, 1985).

cial estimates are that as many as 1.5 million Americans are carrying AIDS antibodies, indicating that they have been "infected" with the disease, even though they may not yet be suffering from the disease itself. Thus, without a crash public health effort, even the conservative figures in the left-hand column indicate that hypothetically the U.S. population could be wiped out by some time between June 1992 and January 1993. The more probable figures on the right (which themselves are, most likely, conservative) indicate an end point between January and June of 1991. In short, if the doubling rate continues, and does not accelerate, the U.S. population has between six and eight years before every American could be infected by a disease which kills everyone who gets it!

DATE	No. of VICTIMS (CDC)	No. of VICTIMS
June 1985	12,000 cases	100,000 cases
Jan. 1986	24,000	200,000
June	48,000	400,000
Jan. 1987	96,000	800,000
June	192,000	1.6 million
Jan. 1988	382,000	3.2 million
June	768,000	6.4 million
Jan. 1989	1.5 million	12.8 million
June	3.0 million	25.6 million
Jan. 1990	6.0 million	51 million
June	12 million	102 million
Jan. 1991	24 million	204 million
June	48 million	No Americans Left
Jan. 1992	96 million	No Americans Left
June	192 million	No Americans Left
Jan. 1993	No Americans Left	

W. J. Hamerman/J. Grauerholz, M.D., FCAP/J. Tennebaum, Ph.D./ D. Freeman, Ph.D./W. Lillge, M.D./N. Roskinsky, M.D./E. Shapiro, M.D./M. Budman/R. Pauls, M.D./C. Cleary/J. Spahn, M.D./B. Kellogg, *Executive Intelligence Report*: "Why Is the Atlanta CDC Covering Up the AIDS Story?" (September 27, 1985), Vol. 12 No. 38.

Disinformation and Distortion

Koop's Glaring Mistakes

AIDS is BIG news and is the most feared disease in the U.S. Americans are confused and suspicious as they hear contradictory statements from different government agencies. Do the AIDS experts agree that there is no possibility of "casual contact"? Is it true that no one has contracted AIDS from a bite, a kiss, or insects? How did a good man like Dr. C. Everett Koop make so many mistakes in his AIDS report (that he agreed to rewrite)? His mistakes are as easy to find as fat lady in a phone booth! What is the truth about AIDS? What do recognized experts like Gallo, Slaff, Seale, Haseltine, Essex, etc. say that are not being reported? One thing is sure: The experts don't agree as we have been led to believe.

Donald Boys, Ph.D., Former member of Indiana House of Representatives

Lack of Information

Senator Don Nickles states, "We are suffering from a severe lack of credible, usable information about the deadliest virus in America."

Joseph Carey/Barbara Quick/Rene Riley, *U.S. News & World Report*: "A Time of Testing: AIDS" (April 20, 1987).

Compromised by Gay Activists

I believe that the Department of Health and Human Services, the Public Health Service, and the Centers for Disease Control have been compromised by "gay" activists and have bent their minds backwards so as not to "offend" homosexuals.

Dr. Paul Cameron, *ISIS Newsletter* (August 1985).

Lobbied by Gay Activists

The major media, with its pro-homosexual bias, is not a reliable source of information. Government officials have been heavily lobbied by "gay" activists. Even the medical establishment has, by and large, been co-opted by the homosexual movement. In fact, opinion-makers in the media, government, and medicine look to the homosexual community as their best source of information about AIDS.

Kirk Kidwell, *The New American* (September 29, 1986), Phoebe Courtney, *The Independent American* (February 1987), No. 217.

Correct Information Could Abort the Epidemic

Dr. June Osborn, Dean of the School of Public Health at the University of Michigan, said that if information of the spread of AIDS were communicated to the public, "We could abort the epidemic."

Paul Raeburn, *News Record*: "Fear of AIDS Strikes Rural Areas" (Associated Press, May 6, 1987).

Media Distorts or Ignores the Truth

We are an amazing nation. Almost daily we are reminded that we are blessed with media analysts who fear nothing and will always tell us the unvarnished truth. Nor do we lightly ridicule the media's sacred cow. Defamation awaits anyone who speaks impiously of, for instance, the Nobel Prize, clubbing seals, Black African governments, Planned Parenthood, anit-Fascists, etc.

With such imperial powers, commentators are tempted now and again to don the Emperor's clothes.

Consider one example. *U.S. News & World Report*, no partisan publication, printed (January 12, 1987) a cover story on AIDS. It exposed the fearful statistics: 29,000 Americans infected, with between 1.5 and four million car-

Dr. Clark, *NFD Journal* (November/December 1987).

Disinformation and Distortion

rying the virus at the end of 1986; by 1991, 179,000 will have died, with 91,000 dying. In twenty years, "a significant portion of our nation may be incapacitated." Dying, that is. AIDS is 100 percent lethal.

With all that, the writers in *U.S. News* danced as close as they dared to the unmentionable fact that promiscuous sodomy is the root cause, not of the untraceable virus, but of incubating the virus into a plague.

U.S. News posed the question bravely. "What causes AIDS?" Answer: "AIDS is caused by a virus usually known as human immuno deficiency virus of HIV." No one laughed. The naked Emperor stared us down. No one in the media dared ask the obvious next question: And how did the HIV get into the bloodstreams of homosexuals who in turn sent it via bisexuals into the bloodstreams of heterosexuals on a plague level?

Remember that these writers are the same men and women who will track apartheid into hidden unconscious prejudice; who will track a national policy to a casual remark of Nancy Reagan; who can trace an anti-Sandinista dollar in and out of Switzerland, Zaire, and the Cayman Islands; who pursue the causes of any social horror — discrimination, censorship, anti-Semitism, fascism — right into the ganglia of miscreants. But our major publications and the networks are satisfied to trace the "cause" of this major death-dealing plague to a dumb, hitherto quiescent virus, not to any human action.

The closest the media came to mentioning real causes is to state that AIDS victims are 65 percent homosexual, 25 percent users of contaminated needles, and four percent heterosexual, with three percent transfusion victims. The unthinking might conclude that AIDS is a disease that comes, with unfair emphases, from many sources — two

Dr. Clark, *NFD Journal* (November/December 1987).

kinds of sex, one needle and one operation. In fact, the virus-turned-plague has only one source — sodomy (primarily anal or rectal sex). Heterosexuals are infected only from homosexuals, or from heterosexuals infected by bisexuals, the latter transmission being impossible without a previous homosexual encounter. Despite the millions of words that have been written on AIDS, this fact is rarely stated.

Dr. Eugene V. Clark, *NFD Journal* (November/December 1987).

Vulgar Gyrations in Front of St. Patrick's Church

Even when the liberated homosexuals go public and put their best foot forward there is still a great deal to be desired. For example, when 50,000 homosexuals marched up Fifth Avenue in New York City under the banner of their "gay flag" (lavender stripes and 50 sex symbols) the lead man had to stop in front of St. Patrick's Cathedral and perform a series of vulgar gyrations. The lesbians and feminists chanted for power, NAMBLA passed out leaflets praising pedophilia, while men and boys walked arm in arm under a banner reading "Man-Boy Love is Beautiful." The Gay militant Atheists chanted: "Smash the state, smash the church, death to the church."

Some chanted: "Pope John Paul, are you gay?"

Others sang: "Two, four, sex, eight, how do you know the Pope is straight?"

When the parade ended in Central Park many of the participants engaged in public sex acts. The gay ideologs, of course, were protected by the pro-homosexual media which showed viewers mostly pictures of ordinary marching bands and two men hugging affectionately.

Dr. David A. Noebel, *The Homosexual Revolution* (Summit Press, Manitou Springs, CO, 1984).

Disinformation and Distortion

Disinformation Campaign
Well-Financed Propaganda

Why do such outlandish things continue? One reason is that there are literally dozens of well-financed organizations working to make AIDS a civil rights issue. These organizations have lawyers and many other professionals as well as being very efficient in the areas of lobbying and propaganda campaigns. It is said that some of them can, with one phone call, marshal millions of dollars for local or national reasons. Where does this money come from? Strangely enough, much of it comes from government grants, some from individual contributions, and enormous amounts from pornographic distributors.

Daily Tribune (July 1987).

(Also, see closing statement of article, entitled "Monkeys and AIDS-Immunization Connection" listed under the heading "Origin of AIDS.")

"Safer Sex" Campaign Exposed as Fraud
How Germany's Dr. Deinhardt Invents
His "Facts" About AIDS

Dr. Friedrich Deinhardt, president of the German Society for the Prevention of Viral Disease, director of the prestigious Max von Pettenkofer Institute in Munich, and leading advisor to the German government on AIDS, is a very peculiar sort of scientist. With almost medieval fanaticism, he insists that only "scientifically proven, hard facts" can be the basis for decisions on AIDS. He rejects all other scientific judgments and hypotheses as "irrelevant" and "mere dreaming."

But closer examination reveals that the chief "scientifically proven facts" cited by Deinhardt in defense of the government's "safe sex" campaign, are pure inventions!

Tennenbaum, *EIR* (April 3, 1987).

Deinhardt admitted this himself in a recent discussion with the author and Dr. John Seale of the Royal Society of Medicine in London. No doubt, Deinhardt wishes to follow in the footsteps of the notorious Francis Bacon, famous for his detailed accounts of the results of experiments which had never been performed.

Unfortunately, if Deinhardt continues unchallenged, his "Baconian" disinformation campaign will cost the lives of hundreds of thousands of persons in West Germany alone who are going to be infected in the coming months as a result of "safe sex" propaganda. This propaganda aims to convince the population that as long as condoms are used, intimate contact with AIDS-infected persons is perfectly safe.

Caught in the Act

During a recent discussion in Deinhardt's Munich office, in the presence of the author and the journalist Jutta Dinkermann, the London doctor John Seale questioned Friedrich Deinhardt on his support for the "safe sex" campaign. Deinhardt, supposedly the leading German authority on AIDS, is caught literally *inventing* a figure of the number of virus particles (the "titer") contained in semen of AIDS carriers. We carry a detailed account of the interchange, since it reveals how very little Dr. Deinhardt really cares about the scientific facts concerning AIDS.

Dr. Seale: How do you think using a condom stops the virus getting across?

Dr. Deinhardt: [With a slight laugh] If the virus is in the semen ...

Seale: What is the titer [amount of virus] in the semen?

Deinhardt: It can be, uh, as far as the studies go, 10SU3, 10SU2, 10SU1 ....

Tennenbaum, *EIR* (April 3, 1987).

Disinformation and Distortion

Seale: Have you got a record of the studies? I would be most interested to read them.

Deinhardt: That is a study which Bob Gallo did. It was reported in Paris.

Seale: Oh, you mean the one with Zagury?

Deinhardt: Yes, But even if it would be 10SU5 or 10SU6, it makes not much difference.

Seale: But, in fact, they did not find *any* virus, except in the lymphocytes, which they had to culture first of all.

Deinhardt: There haven't been more studies? At least, there might have been ...

Mrs. Deinardt [sic]: [Also present] Gallo talked about this again two weeks ago. He didn't talk about titers, but he talked about very high levels.

Seale: Bob Gallo said in the international meeting in Paris, at the plenary session, "We think that the semen is a particularly rich source of virus." Those were his actual words. He also stated in an article in *Nature* that "high titers of cell-free infectuous virions can be obtained from AIDS patients' semen," and gives references which say that they did not even do a titration! Does that not worry you somewhat?

Mrs. Deinhardt: [Very loud] How can *he* [Dr. Deinhardt] answer for Gallo?

Seale: Dr. Deinhart [sic] was at the meeting as well.

Deinhardt: You should write to Bob Gallo and ask him for information, to which study he refers.

Seale: I have done so. So, you are quite happy that there *are* high titers, you said 10SU4, 10SU5 ....

Deinhardt: No, no, no. I said it *probably* would be 10SU3, by analogy with what we see in the serum, what I remember from the studies which were published, although they did not necessarily titrate it, but from the amount of

Tennenbaum, *EIR* (April 3, 1987).

virus they could isolate, the ease with which they could isolate it, and from the amount of virus which was obviously there by electron microscopy. I could not say there could not be *more* [virus in the semen]. I would say probably at least 10SU3.

Seale: [Handing Deinhart [sic] a copy of articles from *Science* magazine in 1984] Here are electron micrographs ....

Deinhardt: That's the paper from Gallo.

Seale: The trouble is, these pictures are of virus in the saliva!

Tennenbaum: There have been no electron micrographs published of AIDS virus in the semen.

Deinhardt: I have seen some, not here but ... I have seen in *Nature* somewhere. [Very irritated] What is the *point*?

Seale: The *facts*, the *facts*, the scientific facts. We have had three papers published on virus in saliva and semen .... And of these three papers, in one they isolated the virus from white cells in the semen from one person after culturing them in T-cell growth factor and Interleukin 2. The other one was of two patients, and they found the virus after culturing the lymphocytes in growth factor for six to seven days. In one paper, they specifically said that they could find no cell-free infectuous virions. But, in the paper on saliva that was published, they grew the virus directly from saliva after passing it through a filter ....

Deinhardt: But I don't see ....

Seale: The technical details are quite important ....

Deinhardt: [Raising his voice] But, Dr. Seale, you want to *get* to something. Why aren't you telling me what you want to *get* to? There is no use talking about technical details. I won't be examined ....

Seale: What I want to know is, *why* is it that you put so much faith in the condom, when nobody has shown that

Tennenbaum, *EIR* (April 3, 1987).

there is more virus in semen or in the vaginal fluid than there is in the saliva? The studies that have been published from the laboratory, show that there is as much or probably more in saliva. How much good is that going to do, if one is wearing a condom in normal sexual intercourse? Nobody has proved, that when the virus is transmitted from husband to wife that the virus went through the semen rather than saliva.

Deinhardt: Because there are a number of studies. I cannot, uh, I am not *willing* to be examined. It is an accepted fact.

Seale: *Why* is it an accepted fact?

The recent discussion in Munich was not the first time Deinhardt had been confronted on the lack of scientific evidence on AIDS transmission by semen. Dr. Seale pointed to exactly the same problem in discussions with Deinhardt and others at an April 1985 conference of the London School of Tropical Medicine and Hygiene. At that time, Deinhardt appeared to be confused on the issue, mistaking an electron micrograph of the AIDS virus in *saliva* for an (apparently nonexistent) picture of virus in the semen. In the intervening nearly *two-year* period, Deinhardt had either not bothered to clarify this crucial matter, or decided to simply *invent* facts as he did in the recent discussion in Munich.

In another part of the Munich discussion, Deinhart [sic] revealed that he is also quite prepared to simply *dismiss* facts which do not fit in with his adopted AIDS policy:

Seale: What do you feel about the study reported in the *Lancet*, from Duesseldorf, about the six-year-old boy who was infected from a three-year-old brother who had a blood transfusion? Do you think the study was wrong? Do you think, in fact, it was sexually transmitted?

Deinhardt: No. I think it is an individual report. There

Tennenbaum, *EIR* (April 3, 1987).

are some things not entirely clear and it is the only report ....

Seale: Just to refresh our memories: The little boy had had a blood transfusion in the first few days of his life; he developed AIDS at the age of 3. Checked back — four donors, one was found to be infected. The mother was not infected, the father was not infected, the brother *was* infected having had no blood transfusion. As a virologist, you must have *some* concept of how the virus got across. It certainly did not come across in the semen.

Deinhardt: The boy had a mark on his arm, though there was no blood.

Seale: So, do you just say it is a mystery? Unexplainable?

Deinhardt: The problem is, I could not talk to the parents or examine the case. I would have had a more *detailed* account of the case than was published in the *Lancet*.

Tennenbaum: Have there been further studies? The boy is in Duesseldorf.

Deinhardt: The doctor was in charge of it, not me. I cannot make any statement when I cannot judge.

Seale: So on the whole, you would prefer not to refer to that case.

Deinhardt: I think it is a case which probably can be dismissed.

A History of Disinformation

The discussion reported above is hardly the first time that Dr. Deinhardt has been caught spreading dangerous disinformation on AIDS.

In January of 1985, the *German Journal of Doctors (Deutsche Aerzteblatt)* published a policy statement on AIDS issued by the German Association for Combatting Virus Diseases, entitled, "AIDS — What Remains After a Critical Examination of the Evidence?" and co-signed by

Tennenbaum, *EIR* (April 3, 1987).

Disinformation and Distortion

Deinhardt himself, states in part: "On the basis of the epidemiology to date and the transmission routes of HTLV-III, a rapid spread of infection by this virus into the general population is not to be expected, and there is no basis for the idea that AIDS represents a new general epidemic acutely threatening the population." The document concludes with the words: "In summary, there is no basis for the supposition of AIDS spread into the general population of the Federal Republic of Germany."

This shameless coverup of the AIDS threat was exposed, soon after its publication, in a letter to the medical journal *Klinische Wochenschrift* by virologist Gerhard Hunsmann and Nobel Prize-winning biochemist Manfred Eigen. Characterizing Deinhardt's play-down of AIDS as "dangerous," the Gouttingen University scientists presented a five-point rebuttal, showing that indeed, there was every reason to fear a spread of AIDS into the general population. They cited the dynamic of the epidemic in the United States, how it spread successively from the group of homosexuals, to blood transfusion recipients, and then into "non-risk" populations. They underlined the great similarity between the AIDS virus and the deadly visna-maedi virus of sheep, and hence the likelihood of a very long incubation period for AIDS. Finally, they pointed out that "the immunological investigation of stored blood transfusion units already indicates an advanced stage of spread of LAV/HTLV-III. In Germany, 1-2 per thousand of stored blood units contain antibody and, most likely, also infectious virus." Hunsmann and Eigen conclude: "The facts reported here speak for themselves." Apparently, Deinhardt simply chose to ignore these facts.

Nearly a year later, in November 1985, the German health ministry of Rita Suussmuth sent out an "information

Tennenbaum, *EIR* (April 3, 1987).

folder" to every household in Germany, which was chiefly designed to counteract the anti-AIDS campaign of the Schiller Institute and the Patriots for Germany. The official brochure reassured the population that catching the AIDS virus was not so dangerous, after all: "Infection does not necessarily lead to getting the AIDS disease. Only 5-15%, at most 20% of infected persons get AIDS." This categorical statement was cooked up out of thin air, without any scientific basis. On the contrary, scientific evidence already existed at the time (and massively confirmed since then) indicates that a very high proportion — perhaps 100% — of infected persons eventually come down with the disease. Again, the leading advisor to the health ministry, Dr. Friedrich Deinhardt, voiced no objection to the cited and other lying statements in the ministry's "information" campaign.

Mass Murder?

How many people are going to die as a result of the continuing campaign of disinformation promoted by Friedrich Deinhardt and other so-called "authorities"? With the partial exception of Bavaria, the health authorities of Germany (and many other countries) have mounted a massive new "information campaign" whose basic message is that sex and other intimate contact with AIDS-infected persons is quite safe, as long as condoms are used; there is no need to know whether your partner is infected or not! Some of this official literature is so explicitly pornographic, that it is becoming the object of litigation by angry parents.

Meanwhile, scientific evidence continues to mount on the transmission of AIDS virus in saliva, by superficial skin injury, insect bites, and aerosols (as in mouth-to-mouth resuscitation). Even if we assume that condoms would be 50% effective in preventing new infection by the AIDS

Tennenbaum, *EIR* (April 3, 1987).

Disinformation and Distortion

virus, failure to enact mass testing and other urgent public health measures will mean that more than 100,000 persons will be newly infected over the coming year in West Germany alone. If the policies recommended by Dr. Friedrich Deinhardt continue to be tolerated, then the chain reaction of infection will reach millions in Germany, tens of millions in Europe, hundreds of millions worldwide.

If humanity survives this holocaust, how will a future Nuremburg Tribunal judge the behavior of "experts" like Dr. Friedrich Deinhardt?

Johnathan Tennenbaum, *EIR* (April 3, 1987).

Doctors With AIDS vs. Patients

Having settled the easy questions about dealing with the AIDS epidemic — Should children with the disease be allowed to attend school? Should condoms be advertised as a protection against contagion? — Americans will soon have to confront the hard ones, such as: Should a doctor with AIDS be allowed to treat patients who are unaware that he is ill?

That question has already presented itself at Chicago's Cook County Hospital. This week the county board voted to keep a physician afflicted with AIDS on staff, while barring him from contact with patients. In doing so, the board rejected the advice of the federal Centers for Disease Control, the hospital's medical staff, and the American Civil Liberties Union, who insist the physician poses no risk to patients.

The medical community appears united on this issue. The CDC guidelines allow doctors to perform all their normal tasks, requiring merely that they take such precautions as wearing gloves during "invasive" procedures — surgery, obstetric examinations, and dental care. The guidelines are based on data that AIDS is transmitted only by such means as sexual intercourse, sharing of contaminated hypodermic needles, and transfusions of infected blood.

End of debate? Not quite. The matter is more complicated than the CDC and its allies presume. In resolving a vexing dilemma, the county board made a prudent choice.

AIDS is a communicable, incurable, and still somewhat mysterious disease. For those reasons — and others, such as its association with homosexuals — it evokes strong aversion. Some of the aversion is baseless, reflecting ignorance. Some of it grows out of uncertainty about the dangers AIDS

Chapman, *Tribune Media Services.*

137

victims pose to those around them.

Doctors may cut themselves accidentally, or they may forget to take the required precautions. Scientists can assure patients of a very high probability that no patient will be infected from the sort of contact that occurs in hospitals. They cannot provide a guarantee. When it comes to an invariably fatal disease, a guarantee is what patients want.

That is not a stupid preference. Hospital patients are routinely exposed to a variety of greater risks — those inherent in anesthesia, some medicines and the diseases carried by other patients — but those risks are unavoidable. More important, they are incurred in exchange for a prospective benefit, namely relief from whatever ailment the patient suffers.

The risk presented by doctors with AIDS may be miniscule, but it is also avoidable: The patient can go to an uninfected physician. There is no necessary trade-off of dangers and benefits. If a patient risks next to nothing from going to a doctor afflicted with AIDS, he may also gain nothing. The natural response of patients is to err on the side of caution.

The medical community would like to prevent that kind of error by denying patients the information needed to make their own choices. When any procedure creates a risk, doctors are obliged to inform patients beforehand. Since the risk here is almost non-existent, they think the information should be withheld.

This extends as far as lying. Dr. George Lundberg, editor of the *Journal of the American Medical Association*, says that if a patient asks an afflicted physician whether he has AIDS, the physician is under no ethical duty to tell the truth.

Surely the correct standard for disclosure is not what the physician deems relevant, but what the patient may find

Chapman, *Tribune Media Services.*

useful. The opposition to providing the information reflects the fear that patients will find it all too useful and will avoid AIDS-infected doctors altogether. The proposed solution is not accurate information, but secrecy. Keeping patients ignorant is supposed to keep them quiescent.

That might work, but it would also undermine public confidence in medical care and medical ethics. It would also relegate patients to the status of children, deprived of the right to make informed decisions about matters affecting their health. In a clash between what patients regard as their well-being and what doctors claim as their prerogative, the interests of patients ought to prevail.

Stephen Chapman, *Tribune Media Services, Inc.* Used by permission.

AIDS Debate Changes Direction

Ira Glasser, the executive director of the American Civil Liberties Union, has regularly proclaimed that "the ACLU sees no conflict between the civil liberties and sound public health policies."

This is nonsense. Consider the following conflict as told to me by a physician during a recent Washington, D.C., meeting of the American Society of Internal Medicine. At the physician's hospital, a surgeon has become infected with the AIDS virus. I asked if his patients are being informed. She shook her head in embarrassment. "We have no policy on that," she said. The surgeon who continued practicing, has, after all, a right to privacy.

Another physician present was appalled. "The duty to warn a patient that he or she may be at risk," he said, "is a compelling ethic." The surgeon in question, however, is now himself a patient and, accordingly, his doctor is prohibited — according to the law of that state — from disclosing the surgeon's infection to anyone without the surgeon's

Hentoff, *The Village Voice* (November 3, 1987).

Doctors

consent.

SO HERE, in collision, are the civil liberties of the infected surgeon and his patients' rights to informed consent not only as to how they're being treated but also as to whether they might be at particular risk from the person who may be treating them.

The patient-doctor privilege creates many more problems with regard to AIDS than the occasional surgeon who may be infectious. The privacy of many other infected patients is also absolutely protected in a number of states. The result is that people who sleep with these patients may be ignorant of the possibility that they, too, might become infected with the AIDS virus.

Few public health officials have been actively concerned about this way of spreading infection with the passive consent of the healing professions. The standard notion is if everyone is educated about AIDS, everyone will practice "safe sex," and the physician-patient privilege can remain intact. If some folks miss the public service ad or pay it no mind, whatever happens to them is their own fault. This country, after all, was built on self-reliance.

In a remarkable change of direction from this myopic view of those who may be exposed to the AIDS virus, Dr. Stephen Joseph, New York City's health commissioner, has broken ranks. He has proposed state legislation that would both add to certain protections of patient confidentiality in AIDS cases and also make clear that doctors and hospitals have a duty, when necessary, to inform the sex partners of patients carrying the AIDS virus that they themselves may now be in danger of becoming infected.

THE PROPOSED bill would safeguard physicians from any liability for having made the disclosure. Current New York state law, like that of a number of other states, forbids

Hentoff, *The Village Voice* (November 3, 1987).

telling sex partners such information without the written consent of the patient.

During a report of Dr. Joseph's testimony at a legislative hearing on AIDS, the *New York Times* included a brief but powerful paragraph that itself was testimony on behalf of the new legislation:

"The city health department says that 1,005 women have contracted AIDS and that many of them did not know their spouses or sex partners were infected."

There is no indication that the ACLU has said anything about the civil liberties of those women.

DR. JOSEPH'S legislation is opposed to the New York State Department of Health. Its officials are still taking the AIDS establishment line that patient confidentiality must not be violated under any circumstances, and that people at high risk will be scared away from doctors and hospitals if they know their sex partners have been told that they test positive.

On the other hand, Dr. Joseph insists that "a physician and a public health authority acting as physician have the ethical obligation and moral duty to issue such a warning when there is a clear risk of infection, even without the explicit consent of the patient."

It is not known yet whether Gov. Mario Cuomo will side with Dr. Joseph's clear medical and ethical imperative or will support the rehearsed responses of his state health department.

At the legislative hearing, two representatives of homosexual rights organizations gave qualified support to Dr. Joseph's proposal and this, too, was a significant change in direction. Said Dr. Joseph: "I'm sure all of us are changing our positions as the epidemic grows. We have to be flexible."

Not all doctors and public health authorities are

Hentoff, *The Village Voice* (November 3, 1987).

Doctors

rethinking their positions. But Dr. Stephen Joseph's decision may have a considerable national impact on the AIDS debate because he is a widely respected member of the AIDS establishment. But he is also, it turns out, an independent member who recognizes there is indeed sometimes a conflict between civil liberties and sound public health policies — and that conflict must be dealt with rather than whistled away.

Nat Hentoff, *The Village Voice*, (New York, NY, November 3, 1987). Used by permission.

Doctors May Keep AIDS Secret
State Panel: Infected Physicians
Need Not Tell Patients

AUSTIN — Texas physicians who test positive for AIDS are not ethically bound to tell their patients, the Texas Medical Association determined Friday.

The disclosure policy, which is identical to the American Medical Association's policy, has generated considerable debate in the Dallas area since September, when it became public through a lawsuit filed by Mesquite pediatrician, Dr. Robert Huse, that he had tested positive for the AIDS virus. Huse subsequently lost nearly all his patients and was forced to sell his practice.

Mesquite resident Debbie McWhorter, whose son was one of Huse's patients, said the medical profession's ethics arbiters should deem it necessary to inform patients when a physician has the AIDS virus or the fatal disease, which breaks down the body's immune system.

"A doctor does have the responsibility to inform us if he carries the AIDS virus," McWhorter contended in comments to the TMA's Reference Committee on Public Health and Scientific Affairs, which held a public forum at the con-

Ard, *Dallas Times Herald* (November 21, 1987).

vention Friday.

McWhorter presented a petition signed by nearly 400 Mesquite residents who favored requiring physicians with AIDS to tell their patients.

"I cannot share with you how agonizing this was," McWhorter said of the day she learned that Huse tested positive for the AIDS antibody. "I feel like he betrayed us. I feel cheated."

The policy on disclosure adopted by TMA officials also stipulates that a doctor who has tested positive for the AIDS antibody "not engage in any activity that creates a risk of transmission...to others," Dougherty said.

It further states that "a physician who has AIDS...should consult with colleagues as to which activities the physician can pursue without creating a risk to patients."

The Board of Governors also adopted a policy calling for doctors to report all AIDS cases to the Texas Department of Health, to provide counseling and to try to persuade the patient not to endanger others. Doctors do not have to inform the spouses of patients who test positive for AIDS, the policy says.

Scott Ard, *Dallas Times Herald* (November 21, 1987). Used by permission.

FDA Drug Bulletin

Precautions for Health Care Professionals

Although HIV is not transmitted through casual contact, the potential for transmission always exists when there is contact with body fluids. Recent reports of transmission of HIV from infected patients to health care workers emphasize the importance of routinely taking all PHS-recommended precautions.

The concentration of virus in body fluids is proportional

Dr. Sherertz, *Medical Clinics of North America* (July 1985).

to the number of white cells in the fluid. Therefore, HIV concentrations are highest in blood and semen, somewhat lower in vaginal secretions, and significantly lower in saliva and tears.

All Invasive Procedures

CDC has published recommended precautions for health care workers involved in invasive procedures. Because the antibody status of most patients will not be known, the recommendations, summarized below, apply to all patients:

All health care workers who perform or assist in invasive procedures must wear gloves when touching mucous membranes or non-intact skin of all patients, and use other appropriate barrier precautions when indicated (e.g., masks, eye coverings, and gowns, if aerosolization or splashes are likely to occur). In the dental setting, as in the surgical and obstetric settings, gloves must be worn for touching all mucous membranes and changed between all patient contacts. If a glove is torn or a needlestick or other injury occurs, the glove must be changed as promptly as safety permits and the needle or instrument removed from the sterile field.

All health care workers who perform or assist in vaginal or cesarean deliveries must wear surgical gloves and use other appropriate barrier precautions when handling the placenta or infant until blood and amniotic fluid have been removed from the infant's skin.

After use, disposable syringes and needles, scalpel blades, and other sharp items must be placed in puncture-resistant containers for disposal. To prevent needlestick injuries, needles should not be recapped, purposefully bent or broken, removed from disposable syringes, or otherwise manipulated by hand.

Dr. Sherertz, *Medical Clinics of North America* (July 1985).

If an incident occurs during an invasive procedure that results in exposure of a patient to the blood of a health care worker, the patient should be informed of the incident, and previous recommendations for the management of such exposures should be followed.

Doctors — Staff Members — Nurses — Orderlies
Precautionary Procedures

Based on this information, the CDC has made certain recommendations for the care of hospitalized AIDS patients. The following precautions should be taken with blood and body secretions:

1. Avoid accidental wounds with sharp instruments used in the care of these patients.
2. Gloves and gowns should be worn when patient specimens may contact personnel or personnel clothing.
3. Label blood and other specimens prominently.
4. Blood and other secretion spills should be cleaned promptly with a disinfectant such as bleach (sodium hypochlorite).
5. All soiled articles and patient waste products should be placed in appropriately labeled plastic bags until they can be disposed of properly or sterilized.
6. A private room is indicated for patients whose secretions or excretions can not be controlled.

Transmission Precautions

Any additional risks of an AIDS patient transmitting an infection are a function of the type of infection that the patient has. For example, if a patient had pulmonary tuberculosis, he would be placed on respiratory isolation in addition to exercising blood and secretion precautions.

Dr. Sherertz, *Medical Clinics of North America* (July 1985).

Doctors

Personnel performing laboratory tests should observe the following precautions:

1. Mouth pipetting should not be allowed.
2. A covering garment should be worn while working with specimens from AIDS patients.
3. Gloves should be worn while handling all specimens.
4. Specimen handling should be carried in a manner that will minimize aerosol generation. Examples of this include capping containers requiring centrifugation and performing procedures at high risk of generating an aerosol (blending, sonication, vigorous mixing) in a biologic safety cabinet.
5. Specimen spills should be cleaned up with a disinfectant, such as bleach (sodium hypochlorite).
6. After processing, all specimens should be decontaminated, preferably by autoclaving, before disposal or reprocessing.

Robert J. Sherertz, M.D., *Medical Clinics of North America* (July 1985), Vol. 69 No. 4.

Doctors of Dentistry, See Dentists

Dried AIDS Virus

Two Weeks

In 1986, Dr. Robert Redfield with the Department of Virus Diseases of the Walter Reed Army Institute of Research wrote a report for Abbot Labs in which he assured them, "The virus is fragile OUTSIDE THE HUMAN HOST (but not internally) and appears to be easily killed by detergents, hand soaps, alcohols, hydrogen peroxide, phenolics, and sodium hypochloride. High and low pH and an exposure to high temperatures will inactivate or kill it."

(Let's see how fragile it really is! — JVI)

Dr. Robert Redfield, Department of Virus Diseases of the Walter Reed Army Institute

Three to Fifteen Days

Infectious cell-free [AIDS] virus could be recovered from dried material after up to three days at room temperature, and in an aqueous environment (e.g. water), infectious virus survived longer than 15 days at room temperature.

L. Resnick, M.D./K. Veren, M.S./S. Z. Salahuddin, MSS/Tondreau, Ph.D./ P. D. Markham, Ph.D., *JAMA — (Journal of American Medical Association)*: "Stability and Inactivation of HTLV-III/LAV Under Clinical and Laboratory Experiments" (1986), Vol. 255 No. 14.

Up to Fifteen Days

The "infectious AIDS-causing virus can live in dried material up to three days at room temperature, up to 15 days in an aqueous environment (e.g. water), and three hours at 133 degrees Farenheit." The AIDS-causing virus can also be present in saliva, tears, semen, vaginal secretions, urine, and feces.

Journal of American Medical Association for 1985

Dried AIDS Virus

Ten Days

A recent report from the Pasteur Institute in Paris by the investigators who originally isolated the lymphadenopathy virus suggests that the AIDS virus might be pretty tough (Lance 1985; I:721-722). The French study finds that the virus survives ten days at room temperature even when dried out in a petri dish.

Charles Marwick, *JAMA — (Journal of the American Medical Association)*: "AIDS-associated Virus Yields Data to Intensify Scientific Study" (November 22-29, 1985), Vol. 254 No. 20.

What Are Your Chances of Getting AIDS From Drugs?

Intravenous drug users who share unsterilized needles are extremely vulnerable. A trace of AIDS-infected blood on a needle or inside the syringe can pass the virus directly into the bloodstream. The user isn't the only one at risk; so is his or her sex partner. This is a major way AIDS is spreading to heterosexuals...and to newborns. Also many prostitutes use needles themselves or have sex partners who shoot drugs.

The Detroit News (January 10, 1988).

Note: It is the infected needle, not the contents that produces death without hope. Throughout this book, one discovers scores of reports indicting drugs by needles. The following world vision release tells the story forcefully. — JVI

Both an international policy statement and a booklet for use by national staff were released this week to leaders in World Vision's 80 offices worldwide.

Seiple said the agency decided to publish the booklet for field staff because it funds and operates many child care, relief and development projects in tropical Africa, where the global epidemic is spreading equally among men and women. A recent report from the U.S. Congressional Select Committee on Hunger estimates that in some African nations one-fourth of all patients have AIDS.

"We have people working in remote areas of the world where it is common practice to use inoculation needles over and over, often without proper sterilization," noted Dr. Rufi Macagba, a Filipino physician responsible for developing the World Vision strategy. Part of the agency's response is to

Dr. Macagba, World Vision International.

Drugs

monitor the sterilization of needles and syringes used in its global program for child survival, which includes inoculating hundreds of thousands of children against common childhood diseases that would otherwise be fatal.

World Vision also will encourage churches to sponsor public AIDS education programs in communities where it worked. In regions where AIDS testing facilities are unavailable, field staff are encouraged to provide testing equipment for local hospitals.

Another suggestion is directed toward staff and church leaders. "We are advising our staff to avoid any inoculations for themselves or their families when comparable oral medicines are available," Dr. Macagba noted. "We also recommend they avoid blood transfusions in places where the blood has not been tested for AIDS infection."

Dr. Macagba also said that traveling staff are being advised to carry disposable syringes with them in case they encounter an emergency while visiting countries where AIDS is widespread.

"Slim disease," as AIDS often is called there because of the weight loss victims suffer, has been estimated to afflict more than 16,000 people in Kampala, Uganda's capital city of 500,000 residents. In Bujumbura, capital of nearby Burundi, one in 10 adults is a carrier of AIDS virus.

Dr. Rufi Macagba, World Vision International

See Section on Vaccinations

Inherited Tendencies a Myth — Seduction the Cause

Dr. Melvin Anchell, medical doctor and psychiatrist, wrote, "Young male children have the characteristics so prized by many male homosexuals." In every television talk show and every debate I have been involved with, this fact is always denied. I am not sure whether my opponents are dishonest or uninformed. Either way, they are wrong.

Anchell continued: "Every homosexual is the product of premature seduction in childhood — regardless of whether the seduction is due to actual attacks by an adult or to overexposure to sexual activities. *All perversions, in fact, are due to interferences in normal sexual development during childhood.* This psychoanalytic conclusion is widely supported by professionals."

Dr. Melvin Anchell, Psychiatrist

Dr. Ralph Slovenko, in his book *Social Behavior and the Law*, reports on his study of inmates imprisoned for sex crimes. Dr. Slovenko concludes that "early sexual experiences have arrested the pervert in an immature state of sexual development, preventing him from making a normal sexual adjustment."

Dr. Ralph Slovenko, *Social Behavior and the Law*

Dr. J. C. Coleman, in his *Abnormal Psychology and Modern Life*, revealed that his discoveries show that half of adult homosexuals have been seduced by older homosexuals before the age of fourteen! And most of those seduced young men never get straight again!

Dr. J. C. Coleman, *The New American*: "Abnormal Psychology and Modern Life" (March 17, 1986).

Homosexuals

When we talk of molestation of children, the tired old knees begin to jerk (the left ones, of course) all over America. But the fact is clear: Homosexuals have perpetrated between a third and a half of all recorded molestations.

Institute for the Scientific Investigation of Sexuality

Almost one year after publication, *The New American* uncovered a startling statement from the Boston-based homosexual publication, *Gay Communcity* [sic] *News*.

Written by the self-described "gay revolutionary," Michael Swift, the statement reads:

"We shall sodomize your sons, emblems of your feeble masculinity, of your shallow dreams and vulgar lies. We shall seduce them in your schools, in your dormitories, in your gymnasiums, in your locker rooms, in your sports arenas, in your seminaries, in your truck stops, in your all-male clubs, in your houses of Congress, wherever men are with men together.

"Your sons shall become our minions and do our bidding. They will be recast in our image. They will come to crave and adore us...

"If you dare cry faggot, fairy, queer at us, we will stab you in your cowardly hearts...All churches who condemn us will be closed. Our only gods are handsome young men...

"We too are capable of firing guns and manning the barricades of ultimate revolution."

Michael Swift, *The New American.*

48% of boys with homosexual experience adopted homosexual habits.

First Kinsey Report

Man's Secret Life Haunts Widow

"No Name" asked you how a woman could tell a homosexual from a bisexual man. Take it from one who knows — there ain't no way!

For 29 years, I was happily married to an attractive professional man. We raised four fine children. He was a great lover, and never did I doubt his loyalty to me. He died suddenly at age 62. When I dismantled his office and opened his safe, all the uglies came spilling out!

He had been an active homosexual since he was 15. I found love letters from Toms, Dicks, and Harrys across the country and Europe. There were canceled checks, proving that for years he had been supporting two guys with generous monthly checks. I found pictures of himself living in two separate worlds — one with his family, the other with his secret companions ranging in age from teens to older men. I was devastated! Not only did this revelation destroy 29 years of beautiful memories, but the embarrassment of feeling humiliated before those who probably knew was worse.

He's been gone for 10 years, and looking back, there were some clues, but at the time I never suspected a thing. If this could happen to me, it could happen to anyone.

The Detroit News: "Dear Abby" (June 18, 1987).

Homosexual Lifestyles

AIDS first appeared in male homosexuals, prompting such initial names as the Gay Compromise Syndrome and Gay Related Immunodeficiency.

Robert J. Sherertz, M.D., *Medical Clinics of North America* (July 1985), Vol. 69 No. 4.

Most people don't know that AIDS was not originally known by that name. In late 1981, it was called "Gay Com-

Source unknown

promise Syndrome," and during the early months of 1982 it was called "Gay Related Immune Deficiency," or GRID. Then on September 3, 1982, the Centers for Disease Control in Atlanta announced a name change — Acquired Immune Deficiency Syndrome (AIDS). This change was made after extensive lobbying by homosexual medical activists.

Source unknown

GRIDS — A Homosexual Originated Disease

Dr. Joseph Sonnabend, a New York City microbiologist, states emphatically that AIDS is a direct result of a homosexual lifestyle. That truth may not be pleasing, but it is correct and nothing can change it.

Dr. Joseph Sonnabend

AIDS in America has always been primarily a disease of male homosexuals.

William Raspberry, *Detroit News* (November 1, 1987).

Sweden took steps to stamp out film and sauna clubs catering to hundreds of homosexual men that the social services say are spreading AIDS.

The Washington Times (March 20, 1987).

AIDS Truth Demands Blunt Words

WASHINGTON — Earnestly, and with applause from journalists, politicians are saying about AIDS: candor, regardless of the cost. But truths are being blurred because they inconvenience a political agenda and shock sensibilities. The agenda is to avoid giving offense to certain factions and to avoid something more terrifying than AIDS — the accusation of "discrimination."

In spite of much talk about the "breakout" into the general heterosexual population. AIDS still is and probably will remain predominantly a disease of homosexuals and intravenous drug users. It will decreasingly afflict educated,

Will, *UPI*

information-receptive homosexuals.

Americans have a technology fixation generally. Regarding health, their thinking is shaped by the polio paradigm, the conquest of disease by Dr. Salk's silver bullet. But America's principal public-health problems flow from foolish behavior regarding eating, drinking, smoking, driving — and, with AIDS, abuse of the body, especially the rectum.

Most journalism about AIDS reflects social and political squeamishness. In addition to an understandable reluctance to discuss certain sexual matters, journalism is infused with liberal values, including abhorrence of "discrimination." That is understood indiscriminately to include all invidious distinctions among social groups, particularly those, such as homosexuals, that have a history of being badly treated.

Journalism seems reluctant to clarify that the primary reason for the AIDS epidemic is that the rectum, with its delicate and absorptive lining, is not suited to homosexual uses. The nation needs unsparing journalism of the sort found in the *Chicago Tribune Magazine* of April 26:

"...81.5 percent of the second cluster of AIDS patients had engaged in the practice called 'fisting,' which causes rectal trauma, in the years before they fell ill. *The researchers defined fisting as the insertion of a portion of the hand — or even the entire fist — into the anus of another person.* The 27 men studied had a median of 120 sexual partners during the year before the onset of symptoms, with one man reporting up to 250 sexual partners in each of the three years before symptoms."

Without here adding details about dildos and enemas, suffice it to say that *the data suggest that receptive anal intercourse is the major, if not the only, important exposure by which homosexuals acquire the infection.* Of course, not all

Will, *UPI*

homosexuals are promiscuous or given to high-risk behavior. (However, even some who are not are dismayed by dissemination of information about those who are). And insufficient information about homosexual practices has impeded understanding of the epidemic.

Time and energy is being wasted on the political project of spreading the false message that the AIDS epidemic is not assignable to particular minorities. British billboards proclaim: "AIDS Doesn't Discriminate," a message designed to absolve homosexuals and addicts of disproportionate responsibility for the epidemic. In New York City, print ads portray a heterosexual couple tangled in sheets, with these words: "Bang, You're Dead!" Such ads are a disservice to the extent that they distract attention from the fact that fewer than four percent of AIDS cases have resulted from heterosexual contact.

Of course anyone with AIDS deserves care and compassion. Of course testing is acceptable, if only marginally important, for applicants for marriage licenses and citizenship, and for prisoners. (Many rapes are homosexual rapes in prison.) But while it is politically safe and socially soothing to pretend that AIDS is now a democratic disease threatening us all equally, that is false.

So is the notion that the most urgent task is to fund research for a vaccine. Of course research should be funded generously, but dollars spent getting addicts off needles and onto methadone will do more good, as will journalism that does not trim the truth to spare our feelings.

George Will, *Washington UPI*

All involved in exposing the vicious homosexual revolution and its venereal disease AIDS know the following comments by Dartmouth professor Jeffrey Hart are abso-

Noebel, *Summit Journal.*

lutely true. *There indeed is a massive cover-up underway and the pro-homosexual media continues to assist the cover-up.*

When the homosexuals were able to take their disease and change its medical name from GRID (Gay Related Immuno-deficiency Disease) to AIDS, one begins to realize their deadly influence. Now the homosexuals are moving heaven and earth to remove themselves from the disease itself.

"American culture," says Jeffrey Hart, "is trying to tell us that AIDS is just the Girl Around the Corner.

"Thus a recent issue of *Newsweek* had a major article on the dread diseases. It began with an AIDS victim called Maria, who was a heterosexual woman, and who had contracted AIDS from a heterosexual man who was a needle user. Practically every case discussed by *Newsweek* was heterosexual, despite what everyone knows — that AIDS at least in North America, is overwhelmingly a homosexual affliction.

"*Newsweek* profiled about a dozen AIDS victims, all of them now dead. Of that dozen, only one, named Robert, was a homosexual. What kind of an editing decision was that?

"*Newsweek*, obviously, is trying to put some distance between AIDS and homosexuality. But for whose benefit?

"For the social benefit of homosexuals, obviously.

"*Newsweek*, is attempting to create the impression that just about anyone can get AIDS, despite the fact that just about anyone is neither a homosexual nor a needle user.

"Obviously, the cultural stakes are high here. Nearly 13,000 people have died of AIDS since statistics on the disease have been kept. In 1995, projections indicate that 10 times that number will die — a plague. The effect on medical insurance and life insurance payments for straight people is going to be, of course, catastrophic. *Newsweek*,

Noebel, *Summit Journal.*

and the rest of our culture, is trying to get the gays off the hook.

"With a reverse spin, we have been told that it is very difficult to contract AIDS. You need to have intimate sexual contact, translated — anal intercourse between men. Now comes a group of honest scientists in Cambridge, Mass., denouncing a New York City study that claimed exactly that. Bad science, say the Cambridge people. Your sample was too small. You rushed to conclusions that are not warranted by the evidence. The AIDS virus, after all, has been discovered in both saliva and tears.

"But why did the New York report venture into bad science and unwarranted conclusions?

"To protect the standing of homosexuals, of course. To prevent food-handlers and hair-dressers from being fired. To let AIDS kids into classrooms — no favor to them, incidentally, since classrooms abound in infections and are a trap for anyone with low-level immune systems.

"The same kind of thing is going on with the blood banks. We are told officially that the nation's blood banks are 'safer than ever.' Only it is not true. Some 400 people now have AIDS as a result of contaminated blood transfusions, and 700 more are being notified that they are at risk after receiving transfusions. Physicians are whispering to their patients the good advice that they establish personal blood banks of their own blood against the possibility of major surgery. You don't want to have your appendix taken out and get AIDS as part of the bargain. But the culture has been covering it up.

"It is interesting that in the *Newsweek* article, the only 'romantic' death is that of the homosexual male, Robert. He dies in the arms of his male lover, who is kissing him and promising to join him soon. Heathcliffe and Cathy in drag.

Noebel, *Summit Journal.*

The heteros who are dying of AIDS are bitter, one woman wishing that the needle-pumper who infected her were still alive so that she could kill him. Yes, he 'cheated death,' by dying, as in the headlines about Hermann Goering's suicide at Nuremburg.

"What is going on here? First, the homosexual culture is powerful enough to affect the way in which it is treated in the media — though not in the scientific journals. Second, the homosexuals have established themselves as a 'victim' and 'minority' category, and we all know how privileged victims are. In fact, established victims are culturally superior. They possess Victim Power.

"In their presence we are all victimized. And truth is a victim."

David A. Noebel, *Summit Journal*

Homosexuals Flex Muscle in Washington

Several hundred thousand homosexual men and women converged on the nation's capital last October for the National March on Washington for Lesbian and Gay Rights, an event hailed by its organizers as "the largest demonstration for gay and lesbian rights in the history of the world."

"We've come to Washington to show our visibility, but also our strength, our anger, our resilience, and our hope," Kay Ostberg, national co-chair of the march, said. "This civil rights movement has come of age politically, and we are not going back to the days of silent suffering. We are here to demand an end to discrimination now."

The march's political tone was set from the start as homosexual activist lobbying teams fanned out across Capitol Hill to meet with Congressmen and Senators.

Saturday October 10 was filled with a hodge-podge of

Kidwell, *AFA Journal* (January 1988).

events, including "The Wedding," in which some 2,000 homosexual couples exchanged "vows." According to its organizers, the event was meant to be a "demonstration for equal rights," not a homosexual marriage ceremony. "The government and heterosexist society has no right to participate in such a celebration," a statement distributed by the march said. "We demand that they stop treating married heterosexuals couples as a privileged class with their laws, their tax structure, and their insurance ratings. If the privileges are not to extend to our families, then they should not exist for theirs."

Later in the day, other activists met at the AFL-CIO headquarters for a "Celebration of Labor Solidarity," honoring "mutual support between the lesbian and gay movement and the U.S. labor movement." In addition, a five-hour Sado-Masachist/Leather conference was held, featuring exhibits of "S & M related [sex] toys and clothing."

The week's activities ended with a civil disobedience demonstration held on the steps of the Supreme Court, resulting in the arrests of more than 600 demonstrators. "Today, we're at the Supreme Court for several reasons. One is to bring our message to the justices of the Supreme Court that gays and lesbians deserve the rights guaranteed all Americans in the Constitution," explained Robin Bray, a march spokesman. "We're here to voice our opposition to the Hardwick decision, and to call attention to the erosion of civil rights toward people with AIDS, AIDS-related complex and HIV-positive individuals." (The Hardwick decision was a 1986 Supreme Court decision upholding Georgia's anti-sodomy law.)

The main event of the week, however, occurred on Sunday October 11 as an estimated 200,000 to 300,000 homosexuals marched from the Ellipse, past the White House, to the

Kidwell, *AFA Journal* (January 1988).

Capitol. "We are here today to show America and the world that the gay movement is larger, stronger, and more diverse than ever," proclaimed Buffy Dunker, an 82-year-old lesbian who "came out of the closet" 10 years ago. "We are sending a message to our leaders here in Washington that gays are a united force that will have to be reckoned with. And we will be persistent and unrelenting in our pressure."

National activist organizations like the National Gay Rights Advocates, the Gay and Lesbian Task Force, the Lambda Legal Defense Fund, and the Human Rights Campaign Fund were intermingled with local homosexual groups from across the nation. Religious homosexual organizations were represented as well, including Dignity, Integrity, the Unitarian Universalist Association, the United Church of Christ, and the homosexual Universal Fellowship of Metropolitan Community Churches.

Marchers carried signs and banners, which proclaimed: "Thank God, I'm Gay"; "Our Bedrooms Are None of Your Business, Abolish Sodomy Laws"; "Get Ready for the Gay 90's"; and "Condoms, Not Condemnation." Another sign carried by two leather-clad marchers read, "Diversity is American." The chants were as varied as the signs: "Two, Four, Six, Eight, Aren't You Glad You're Not Straight"; "We Are Everywhere, California to Delaware"; "What Do We Want? Gay Rights! When Do We Want It? Now!"; "Money for AIDS, Not for War."

The march ended with a rally at the Capitol, featuring a keynote speech by Democratic presidential candidate Jesse Jackson. "We gather today to say that we insist on equal protection under the law for every American, for workers' rights, women's rights, for the rights of religious freedom, the rights of individual privacy, for the rights of sexual preference. We come together for the rights of all American

Kidwell, *AFA Journal* (January 1988).

people." Noting that he had just officially declared his presidential candidacy the day before the rally, Jackson ended his speech by urging: "Today I stand with you, Election Day you stand with me."

Other speakers at the rally included two homosexual members of Congress, Representatives Gerry E. Studds and Barney Frank, both Democrats from Massachusetts; Eleanor Smeal, former president of the National Organization for Women; leftist labor leader Cesar Chavez; and actress Whoopi Goldberg and actor Robert Blake.

Kirk Kidwell, *The AFA Journal* (January 1988).

500,000 in D.C. Demand
Lesbian/Gay Rights Now

The above caption appeared in the October 22 edition of *Workers World*, a communist weekly, published in New York.

The unprecedented gall of the homosexual community is staggering. The unbridled indulgence in sodomy by consenting adults is the cause of the AIDS plague which is bringing torment and death to thousands. Nevertheless, they demand the right to continue to indulge in this disease-spreading practice.

Many of the victims of AIDS have contracted the disease from transfusions of AIDS-infected blood. They include hemophiliacs and people undergoing surgery. Most were infected before the blood used in transfusions was tested or the AIDS virus, as is now the case.

In addition to male homosexuals, many drug addicts, who share needles, are infected. These in turn have produced infected babies. The tragic sequence is devastating, and it is unbelievable that any sane person could demand the right to perpetuate it.

Dr. Swartz, *Anti-communist Crusade*

Despite this, one of the objectives of the marchers was to secure the abolition of all laws prohibiting sodomy between consenting adults in private. This is a demand for the right to continue to spread AIDS. Words fail! Madness rules!

Dr. Swartz, M.D., *Anti-communist Crusade,* Vol. 27 No. 22.

The press on occasion seems almost oversolicitous of high risk groups because most reporters don't have much of an understanding of the GAY COMMUNITY. THEY OFTEN GET VERY NERVOUS AND DON'T WANT TO OFFEND (GAYS).

Newsweek (September 23, 1985).

Henry Waxman: The Bodyguard of Homosexuals

AIDS, potentially the most serious health catastrophe since the Black Death of the Middle Ages, could, some experts say, wipe out a quarter of the world's population by the end of this century.

The obvious response to such a disaster is to attempt, as far as possible, to contain the spread of the disease. That calls for identifying those who are infected and preventing them from infecting others, accidentally or intentionally.

This would be a routine matter with any other disease: the bubonic plague, typhoid, measles. But AIDS is different. It is 1) incurable, 2) deadly, and 3) it was introduced and became an epidemic through homosexual promiscuity.

The first two factors make AIDS frightening. The last one makes it history's first politically protected disease.

Among its chief protectors is Rep. Henry Waxman, the California Democrat who runs the House Subcommittee on Health and Environment.

Waxman has used his position to keep any effective AIDS-containment measures from being considered and to

Liberty Report (November 1987).

steer the congressional debate, as far as possible, away from protecting the uncontaminated and towards protecting the already infected.

Waxman's antagonist is another member of the Health and Environment Subcommittee; Congressman from Southern California Bill Dannemeyer has been waging a valiant effort to get Congress to face the AIDS crisis and protect public health.

He has sponsored eight bills on the subject, all of which are languishing in Waxman's subcommittee with no hearing, no votes, and no official mention of them. As far as Waxman is concerned, the Dannemeyer bills can stay in the subcommittee's "in" box until all the seas run dry.

The subjects covered by Dannemeyer's bills provide a good summary of what needs to be done to protect public health in the face of the AIDS plague:

Reportability. Infection with the AIDS virus should be reportable to public officials. This is the only way the spread of the disease can be tracked.

Testing. Routine testing of as many people as possible will enable public health officials to localize the spread of AIDS infection. Most people with AIDS do not even realize they are infected. Many who suspect that they may have AIDS do not want to be tested, preferring to remain ignorant to change their behavior patterns.

Requiring the testing of persons in sensitive occupations (health care, food preparation) or in high-risk groups (prostitutes, drug addicts, prison inmates) or capable of infecting others (blood donors, marriage license applicants) is an effective means of reducing the spread of the disease and directing public health efforts to where they are most needed.

Protection. Health care and emergency personnel should

Liberty Report (November 1987).

have the right to take precautions to minimize their chances of contracting AIDS.

Sanctions. Members of high-risk groups should not be donating blood or organs. Transmission of the disease should be a criminal offense. Persons with AIDS should not be employed in jobs where they might infect others.

On all of these issues, Dannemeyer's bills represent not only common sense, but the overwhelming consensus of public opinion on what should be done to halt the spread of AIDS.

If these measures were adopted, it might not become necessary to resort to a quarantine of infected persons. Yet none of it is happening because Henry Waxman has an agenda of his own.

He is well aware that serious action to stop the spread of AIDS will eventually call into question the legitimacy of promiscuous homosexual behavior. That, after all, is how AIDS became a plague; and, even now, it remains the main vector of transmission.

No matter how sensitive one is to the feelings of gay militants, any serious campaign against AIDS is going to have to make it clear that no one has a right to endanger lives by committing random sodomy with strangers.

That is the real reason why Waxman is sitting on the Dannemeyer legislation and preventing these remedies from even being discussed in hearings. He has yet to unveil his own package of AIDS legislation.

He has, however, let it be known how he thinks the AIDS crisis should be met.

Reportability is absolutely out for Waxman. He fears that public health officials cannot be trusted to maintain the ordinary standards of medical confidentiality and might make public the identity of AIDS carriers, thus subjecting

Liberty Report (November 1987).

Homosexuals

them to harassment and discrimination.

For the same reason, he says testing must be offered only on a voluntary basis and the results must be kept in the strictest secrecy, lest AIDS carriers be "stigmatized."

The other measures Dannemeyer has proposed are, in Waxman's eyes, nothing but "gay-bashing." Even granting health care workers the right to wear protective clothing or to know that they are treating a person with AIDS is viewed as discriminatory.

After all, he says, there have been only a few recorded instances of AIDS transmission to nurses or dentists, and protecting them is not worth inflicting embarrassment or mental unease on AIDS carriers.

The positive measures Waxman favors center essentially on awarding huge federal grants to gay rights groups to carry on "educational" campaigns. He wants to extend civil rights laws so that the condition of having AIDS will be placed on the same level as belonging to a minority race.

AIDS carriers, in Waxman's scenario, would be assured the right to hold any job, regardless of the possibility of exposing others to the disease; the right to marry and/or adopt children; the right to mix freely with persons not yet infected in prisons and military installations; the right to donate blood and to have sexual relations with the not-yet-infected.

In short, Waxman is regarding AIDS less as a problem than an opportunity to smuggle in the most extreme goals of the gay rights movement under the guise of protecting the "handicapped" from discrimination.

AIDS infection is not limited to homosexuals, but it is overwhelmingly concentrated among those who habitually engage in homosexual practices.

Unless protective measures are undertaken, it is simply a

Liberty Report (November 1987).

matter of time before virtually all active homosexuals will be infected; and of course, as the disease becomes more wide-spread among homosexuals, it will also expand among those elements of the population who do not indulge in "high-risk" activities.

It is perfectly evident that Waxman's approach to the AIDS crisis will lead to broadening AIDS infection and eventually to millions of additional deaths. Yet this appears to be preferable, in his estimation, to the alternative.

He knows that serious protective measures that approach AIDS as a public health issue instead of as a civil rights issue will inevitably entail speaking out against homosexual prac-tice — a fate too horrible to contemplate.

Liberty Report (November 1987).

Moral Americans Must Counter Homosexual Lobby — Homosexuals Protected

The homosexual lobby has been actively pressuring Sena-tors and Congressmen from all fifty states to oppose any bill they consider "anti-gay." A day rarely passes in most Cap-itol Hill offices without a postcard or letter from a member of a pro-homosexual group. An aide to one Senator states that over thirty postcards and letters have arrived against AIDS testing by insurance companies alone.

Most Senators and Congressmen try to vote the way the majority of those they represent wish them to. Unless they hear from people like you, they think only the homosexuals care about these issues and will vote as they ask them to.

Right now, the House of Representatives must decide whether or not to support Congressman William Danne-meyer's bill to repeal the Supreme Court's decision that contagious disease carriers cannot be "discriminated" against. Senator William Armstrong has introduced a sim-

Action Alert, Liberty Foundation.

ilar repeal bill in the Senate.

The Armstrong and Dannemeyer bills are just two of many homosexual-related bills your Senators and Congressmen will be debating this year. The 60 votes we lost from last year to this in the House indicate the Congress is hearing from the gay lobby.

Action Alert, Liberty Foundation.

Protesters

We have a sick public health community that has been frankly intimidated by the homosexual lobby.

Paul Weyrich, *Time* (March 23, 1987).

Scandal

Why Should We Pay To Teach Gays Safe Sex?

WASHINGTON — On May 1, 1986, the National Centers for Disease Control made a grant of $239,962 in public funds to the Gay Men's Health Crisis Inc. of New York. This May the grant was renewed for another $434,717, making a total of almost $675,000 for the two years.

U.S. taxpayers often wonder what in the world the government does with their money. The two grants are instructive. They tell us something about how our nation has run up a debt of $2 trillion. These particular dollars were poured out in an effort to promote safe sodomy among male homosexuals.

The story came to light last month when Sen. Jesse Helms, R-N.C., offered an amendment to a pending appropriation bill. The senator's purpose was to put a halt to outlays for this purpose. After a spirited debate, in which Sen. Lowell Weicker, R-Conn., "yelled" (his verb) his opposition to any such restriction, the amendment passed

Kilpatrick, *Detroit Free Press* (November 17, 1987).

by a vote of 94-2. The other opposing vote came from Sen. Daniel Patrick Moynihan, D-N.Y.

The Gay Men's Health Crisis Inc. proposed to spend the $675,000 in part on a manual for conducting "Eroticizing Safer Sex Workshops." These workshops, according to the grant application, are intended to help participants "discover and share information on how to be sexually active in low-risk ways." Another purpose is to help participants "improve levels of sexual functioning." This is "education"?

Under the approved program, workshops are to be divided into sessions. The first session is "therapeutic." It is intended to console homosexuals who are "mourning the loss of old sexual partners and the loss of being able to act on the sexual impulse."

A second session is to be devoted to "affirming that a wide variety of sexual options is open to them."

In a third session, participants are to discuss how to "eroticize" safer options. In a fourth, they are to learn "how to negotiate safer sex agreements." All sessions are to be led by a moderator who is "unconditionally sex-positive." His task is to "dispel the myth that normal heterosexuality is superior to homosexuality"....

How can such frivolous grants be justified? Even Weicker acknowledged that "there is no better educated community than the homosexual community." If these people haven't heard about "safe sex" by this time, no happy little workshops will teach them.

James J. Kilpatrick, *Detroit Free Press* (November 17, 1987). Used by permission of Universal Press Syndicate.

Death Sentence of AIDS
Long Incubation Period

The evidence that the AIDS-associated retrovirus can be classified as a lentivirus is overwhelming. Clinical findings that are characteristic of both the lentivirus and ARV are the association with a disease with a long latency period...

J. A. Levy, M.D./L. S. Kaminsky, M.D./W.J.W. Morrow, Ph.D./K. Steimer, Ph.D./P. Luciw, Ph.D./D. Dina, M.D./J. Hoxie, M.D./L. Oshiro, Ph.D., *Annals of Internal Medicine*: "Infection by the Retrovirus Associated with the Acquired Immunodeficiency Syndrome."

Death Sentence of AIDS
Ten to Fifteen Year
Incubation Period

...viruses are known to incubate 10 to 15 years before causing illness.

Dr. Dean Echenbert, *San Francisco Examiner* (November 29, 1985), p. 1.

Infected for Life

It now appears that all persons who have been infected with the AIDS virus will remain infected for life, probably capable of being infectious to others.

Dr. Paul Kaldahl, *Special Report: AIDS* (Noebel/Lutton/Cameron), p. 52.

No Hope

After listening to 1,238 scientific reports at the Third International Conference on AIDS, the largest AIDS meeting ever held,...it is becoming increasingly clear that most people who are infected with the AIDS virus will ultimately get AIDS or a related disease.

"That's really sad news," said Peter Piot of the Institute of Tropical Medicine in Belgium. "There is no evidence of slowing down of [sic] incidence over the years."

Star Tribune: "AIDS Epidemic Outpaces Research, Agency Says" (Associated Press, June 7, 1987), p. A-11.

Underestimating Carriers

Ingram stated, "They have been underestimating, I think, the proportion of people that carry the disease and...the speed at which (those people) are going to get AIDS."

Star-Tribune: "AIDS Insurance Cost to Hit $50 Billion, Study Says" (Associated Press, August 5, 1987), p. B-9.

Death Strikes San Francisco

In San Francisco, which has the second largest number of cases after New York,...all of the patients who contracted AIDS three years ago, and 75 percent of those who have contracted it in the last two years, are dead.

Peter Collier/David Horowitz, *California Magazine*: "Whitewash" (July 1983).

Twenty-two Million Dead Americans

We are in the very early stage of what all evidence indicates may be a terrible world-wide epidemic, possibly killing 10 percent of the population or more. AIDS may kill 22 million Americans in the next few years. What we have to do, and quickly, is to get our people and more specifically our young people to change their sexual behavior. Promiscuity is a certain way to get infected with HTLV-III. Our young people especially need to know this.

Ronald K. Wright, M.D., Chief Medical Examiner, University of Miami School of Medicine, Dr. Ed Rowe, *CMA Newsletter*.

Expert: AIDS Top Young-Male Killer by '91

LONDON — AIDS will become the No. 1 killer of young men in the West by 1991, an expert predicted Tuesday at the first world summit on the deadly disease.

The expert, Dr. Johnathan Mann, U.S. director of the World Health Organization's Special Program on AIDS,

Drs. Wright, Rowe, *CMA Newsletter*.

estimated that the number of AIDS cases worldwide will reach one million in three years and that by 1991 in the West, the disease will surpass the combined total of the current top-four leading causes of death in men between the ages of 25 and 34: traffic accidents, suicides, heart disease, and cancer.

"We do not have precise numbers, but it is likely that several hundred million people around the world may have behaviors which make them potentially vulnerable to infection with HIV," the virus that causes AIDS, he said.

Acquired immune deficiency syndrome weakens the body's immune system and is fatal. The virus that causes it is spread most commonly through sexual contact or the sharing of hypodermic needles by drug users.

The disease also is transmitted from mother to fetus through the bloodstream before birth or during birth through contact with the birth canal.

Britain's Princess Anne, in the opening address at the summit, told delegates that AIDS was a profound tragedy that man had brought upon himself.

Scrapping her prepared text in favor of stronger language, the queen's daughter said, "The global response to AIDS has been characterized by a series of delays.

"World summits are not quick or easy to organize and don't always produce results. Please make this one work. Make this summit be the forerunner of the most genuine international cooperation ever seen."

The Detroit News (January 27, 1988) p.3-A.

"It's my job to take care of patients unable to breathe on their own, without the help of a machine — in other words, the dying AIDS patients. You see these young people come in and die so quickly and in such agony. Their family comes

Collier/Horowitz, *California Magazine* (July 1983).

in and watches. It's terrible when parents outlive their children...It's horrible. And it's a horrible death. The patients waste away until they look like Dachau victims in the end. I see all this happen, and I have to admit that some of those responsible are gay leaders. In my mind they're criminally negligent. They've betrayed their own community."

Peter Collier/David Horowitz, *California Magazine*: "Whitewash" (July 1983), p. 57.

Origin of AIDS

In my introduction of this work I stated that this book would be a secular rather than religious presentation. At this point, however, I would like to include an article I find shocking concerning a disease similar to AIDS recorded centuries ago in the Holy Bible. — JVI

AIDS Is Not a New Disease

Dr. Robert W. Feldtman is a Clinical Assistant Professor of Surgery at the University of Texas Health Science Center in Houston. He is also a Lt. Col. in the U.S. Air Force Reserves. Recently he released his thoughts regarding the AIDS plague and the Bible. Since he works with AIDS patients his reflections take on even deeper significance. He says, "In II Chronicles 21:12 we are told, 'And a letter came to him from Elijah the prophet saying,

'Thus says the Lord God of your father David: Because you have not walked in the ways of Jehosophat [sic] your father or in the ways of Asa King of Judah, but have walked in the ways of the Kings of Israel and have made Judah and the inhabitants of Jerusalem to play the harlot like the harlotry of the house of Ahab and have also killed your brothers those of your fathers household who were better than yourself, behold the Lord will STRIKE YOUR PEOPLE WITH A SERIOUS AFFLICTION — YOUR CHILDREN, YOUR WIVES, AND ALL YOUR POSSESSIONS: AND YOU WILL BECOME VERY SICK WITH A DISEASE OF YOUR INTESTINES, UNTIL YOUR INTESTINES COME OUT BY REASON OF THE SICKNESS, DAY BY DAY.

'After all this the Lord struck him in his intestines with an incurable disease. Then it happened in the course of time AFTER TWO YEARS THAT HIS INTESTINES CAME OUT BECAUSE OF HIS SICKNESS SO HE DIED IN

Dr. Feldtman, *The Independent Baptist Voice* (November 5, 1987).

174

SEVERE PAIN...He was thirty-two years old when he became king. He reigned in Jerusalem eight years and, to no one's sorrow, he departed.' "

From a medical standpoint this accurately describes the end stages of AIDS. The patient first starts out with the "gay-bowel" syndrome. Because of the destruction of the immune system, and the frequent oral-anal contact between homosexual partners, parasitic and bacterial diseases flourish in the intestines of homosexual males. Amebic dysentery is very common among this group, and bacterial diarrheas occur as well. In the end stages of an AIDS patient his care becomes very complex. Massive amounts of fluid and electrolyte loss from stool have to be replaced by intravenous electrolyte solutions.

Such a condition is obviously messy and requires constant nursing attention.

Ironically, public health officials in the U.S. continue to support "gay rights" to work in food establishments even with known, diagnosed AIDS. They argue that AIDS can't be transmitted by fecal contamination of food, but they are strangely silent about the the transmission of other parasitic, viral, and bacterial diseases that are (ameba, hepatitis, bacterial diarrheas).

Elihu's comments to Job about God — in Job 36:6,13 & 14, "He does not keep the wicked alive but gives the afflicted their rights.

"The godless in heart harbor resentment, even when he fetters them they do not cry out for help.

"They die in their youth, among the male prostitutes of the shrines."

Those who think AIDS is a new disease better think again. It is as old as the sin of homosexuality. The virus has just reared its ugly head because of the rampant immorality of

Dr. Feldtman, *The Independent Baptist Voice* (November 5, 1987).

the Western world. It is as destructive to the immune system and the nervous system as syphilis is to the blood vessels and brain or alcohol is to the liver and brain....

[Let's continue.]

:21 — "The Lord will make the plague cling to you until He has consumed you from the land which you are going to possess.

:22 — "The Lord will strike you with consumption, with fever, with inflammation, with severe burning fever,...until you perish.

:27 — "The Lord will strike you with the boils of Egypt, with tumors, with the scab, and with the itch, from which you CANNOT BE HEALED.

:28 — "The Lord will strike you with madness, and blindness and confusion of the heart.

:35 — "The Lord will strike you in the knees and on the legs with severe boils which CANNOT BE HEALED and from the sole of the foot to the top of the head.

:59 — "Then the Lord will bring you and your descendants extraordinary plagues — great and prolonged plagues — and serious and prolonged sicknesses.

:60 — "Moreover He will bring back on you all the diseases of Egypt, of which you were afraid, and they shall cling to you.

:61 — "Also every sickness and every plague which is not written in the book of this law, will the Lord bring upon you until you are destroyed."

Today two million to three million Americans have the antibody to the AIDS virus. Liberal doctors say that only means the patients were "exposed" to the virus. Another test, the AIDS antigen test has just been developed, and the great majority of AIDS antibody positive patients also test positive for the antigen, therefore they have AIDS, and

Dr. Feldtman, *The Independent Baptist Voice* (November 5, 1987).

therefore they are infective. Dr. Joseph, the public health official in New York City, estimates that one out of ten adults in New York City, are antibody positive.

Since 10 to 15 years may be needed to allow the full presentation of the disease, it is easy to see how easy some conservatives are concerned that hundreds of thousands of Americans are destined to die, possibly millions.

Tuberculosis, once thought to be under control in the U.S. has had an eruption of outbreaks in the homosexual community. Almost all AIDS patients have it. Many ARC (AIDS-Related Complex) patients have TB. The old description of TB is consumption, as noted above in the Bible passages.

The Bible states that "madness" will ensue. Realize that the AIDS virus zeroes in on the central nervous system, and sets up house there. The brain is slowly destroyed and AIDS encephalopathy causes madness. The patient slowly becomes a sociopath.

Dr. Robert W. Feldtman, Professor of Surgery, University of Texas, Health Science Center in Houston, *The Independent Baptist Voice* (November 5, 1987).

Kaposi's Sarcoma — Associated With AIDS Is Not New — It Was Discovered in 1872

Histopathology of Kaposi's Sarcoma and Other Neoplasms

In 1872, Moris Kaposi, the renowned Viennese dermatologist, described a disease that now bears his name. He initially termed the entity "Multiple idiopathic hemorrhagic sarcoma". In his original description the disease [was] presented as red-blue nodules predominantly on the lower extremities. The 3 patients described were all adult males and died within 3 years of diagnosis. Histologically the

Source unknown

lesions exhibit proliferation of vessels, hemorrhage, and hemosiderin pigment deposition. For over half a century after Kaposi's original description, the literature was mainly concerned with the clinical and pathologic aspects of the disease and its epidemiology in Europe, especially in Eastern European (Ashkenazic) Jews.

The past three decades have seen remarkable and rather startling epidemiologic and etiologic observations in this previously rare disorder. An increased prevalence of Kaposi's sarcoma (KS) was noted in Equatorial Africa. A compilation of the work of many investigators on this subject is found in a monograph published after a symposium on KS which was held in Kampala, Uganda in 1961.

The next important epidemiologic observation consisted of reports of KS in patients with immunodeficient states either due to immunodeficient disorders such as lupus erythematosus or as a result of immunosuppressive therapy such as kidney transplant recipients.

In the past 3 years an outbreak of KS appearing mostly in homosexual males has been observed. The term Acquired Immunodeficiency Syndrome (AIDS) has been coined to define this entity that, although most commonly seen in homosexual males, is also seen in IV drug abusers, hemophiliacs, and Haitians. KS associated with AIDS is frequently complicated with opportunistic infections such as *Pneumocystis carinii* pneumonia.

Source unknown

In 1981 Kaposi's Sarcoma Resurfaces

In June 1981, Atlanta's Centers for Disease Control published what was to be the first report on the strange new ailment.

No sooner did the report appear than the CDC began

Time Magazine (August 12, 1985).

hearing from doctors in San Francisco and New York City, who were also seeing PCP in young homosexual men. And that was not all they were seeing. Many of the patients bore the purplish lesions of Kaposi's sarcoma, a rare skin cancer that in this country is usually found only in elderly men of Mediterranean extraction. They had other infections as well: *Candida albicans*, a fungus that cakes the mouth and throat, making it difficult and painful to speak or eat; herpes, not just the garden variety of sores, but ulcerating infections of the mouth, genitals, or anus that raged for months. The patients fell prey to exotic bugs seen more often in animals than humans, like *Toxoplasma gondii* and *Cryptosporidium*, which causes diarrhea. Doctors were appalled. Says Dr. Paul Volberding, 36, who heads the AIDS clinic at San Francisco General Hospital, "You see someone your own age dying of such a gruesome disease that you can't do anything to stop."

By late August, less than three months after its initial report, the CDC knew of more than 100 cases of what was already being called the gay plague ... What they had in common was something Gottlieb observed in the first four cases, "a near wipe-out" of helper T cells, a class of white blood cells that plays a central role in orchestrating the body's immune defenses.

As the mystery deepened and the number of cases rose, the CDC intensified its investigation into the causes of the syndrome. Disease detectives interviewed scores of homosexuals about their sexual practices to test the hypothesis that AIDS was somehow tied to the gay life-style. They briefly considered and then discarded a theory linking AIDS to the use of "poppers" (liquid inhalants like amyl nitrite and butyl nitrite), which are said to enhance sexual pleasure and which had been used by many of the victims. Another

Time Magazine (August 12, 1985).

theory held that repeated anal intercourse introduced sperm into the bloodstream and that this could cause profound immune suppression. Then there was the "immune-overload theory," which was based on the fact that many early AIDS patients were extremely active sexually, with hundreds of partners over the course of their lifetimes and long histories of venereal diseases and infections. Under the accumulated burden of so many infections, the overload theory suggested, their immune systems had simply given up.

But most of these explanations were abandoned as evidence grew that AIDS was caused by an infectious agent that could be passed from one person to another through sexual contact or in body fluids. The evidence included a "cluster" of nine patients in and around Los Angeles; each had had sex with people who later developed AIDS-related diseases. It was bolstered by the growing number of intravenous drug users infected by the disease. Addicts share germs when they share needles. Then came the clincher: cases of AIDS in hemophiliacs and later in recipients of donor blood. The pattern resembled that of hepatitis B, a blood-borne and sexually transmissible virus that is common among drug addicts, blood recipients, and gay men. AIDS cases among Haitian men and women remained a puzzle until it was discovered that many of the men, though not homosexually inclined, had warded off destitution by serving as prostitutes to gay men. Earlier this year, Haitians were dropped by the CDC as a separate risk category for AIDS.

Are Monkeys Responsible?

The virus apparently appeared in the late 1970's, when monkeys at the Harvard-run center began to die from a mysterious affliction that scientists now say bore remarkable similarity to AIDS ... The Harvard scientists do not know how the virus was introduced into the monkey colony nor how the virus spread among monkeys, but they note that the animals formerly lived in group cages where heterosexual and homosexual relations, the eating of feces, and the spraying of urine were frequent. The incidence of the simian disease at the center has declined since the monkeys were rehoused in individual cages.

Erik Eckholm, *The New York Times*: "AIDS-like Ailment Given to Monkey" (September 27, 1985).

From Monkey to Man

Dr. Myron Essex, of Harvard School of Public Health, says that 42% of a group of healthy green monkeys had blood that indicated an AIDS infection. The green monkey has more contact with humans than do other primates, and it is suggested that the AIDS virus leaped from monkey to man (as yellow fever did) through bites, scratches, ingesting the flesh, or sex with monkeys.

Dr. Myron Essex, Harvard School of Public Health

Testing Monkeys

Dr. Robert Gallo, head of a U.S. National Institutes of Health (NIH) team that provided convincing evidence of the AIDS link, says if there is not a vaccine that works in chimpanzees by the end of this year, "I'll be very worried." Even then, it would take several years for the vaccine to be proved out.

Dr. Robert Gallo, U.S. National Institutes of Health, *Reader's Digest* (June 1987).

Origin of AIDS

The Culprit

But what about the green monkey? Some of the best virologists in the world and many of those directly involved in AIDS research, such as Robert Gallo and Luc Montagnier, have said that the green monkey may be the culprit.

U.S. National Institutes of Health

Relative of AIDS Virus May Spread, Hurting Vaccine Bid

BOSTON — A lethal relative of the AIDS virus is likely to spread from Africa to the rest of the world, which could seriously complicate the already-difficult job of finding an AIDS vaccine, researchers say.

The microbe, HIV-2, also could raise questions about the accuracy of AIDS tests.

HIV-2, discovered in 1984, genetically resembles HIV-1, the virus that causes AIDS found in the United States, and SIV, the virus that causes an AIDS-like disease in monkeys.

Atlanta Journal (May 7, 1982) p. 24.

More Monkey Business: New Epidemic Feared From Cousin of AIDS Virus

BOSTON — A cousin of the AIDS virus found in west Africa causes a disease indistinguishable from AIDS and may spread to ignite a new AIDS epidemic, French researchers say.

The virus, called HIV-2, was discovered in 1984. It is distinct from HIV-1, which causes AIDS in the United States, Europe, central Africa and other parts of the world.

"It seems to be localized at the moment" in west Africa, said Dr. Francois Clavel of the Pasteur Institute. "But there is no reason why this epidemic would not spread over Africa

Dallas Morning News (May 7, 1987).

or Europe or other countries like HIV-1 did, unless we are very vigilent [sic] and can detect carriers of the virus.''

Earlier, researchers from the Pasteur Institute in Paris reported finding HIV-2 in two AIDS patients. Clavel said the latest study, documenting HIV-2 infection in 30 people, provides strong evidence that the virus actually causes the disease.

Though genetically different, the two viruses appear to attack the body in similar ways and cause identical disease. However, the differences between the two microbes could complicate efforts to find an AIDS vaccine.

The researchers studied HIV-2 infection in 30 people from Guinea-Bissau or the Cape Verde Islands who were treated in Lisbon. Of these, 17 had acquired immune deficiency syndrome; the rest had AIDS-related complex or no symptoms. None of them was infected with HIV-1.

In their report, published in Thursday's *New England Journal of Medicine*, the French researchers wrote that ''it appears clear the HIV-2, a virus related to but distinct from HIV-1, is the cause of AIDS in some west Africans and that a new AIDS epidemic is possible (but not yet documented) in west Africa.''

Clavel said that while some parts of HIV-1 and HIV-2 are genetically alike, others are different, and the overall genetic similarity is about 40 percent.

Because of this, he said, the standard screening test used to check blood for AIDS will often miss the HIV-2 virus. So these tests, at least when used in Africa, should be modified to include sensitivity to HIV-2.

Clavel said it is unclear what, if any, significance the emergence of a second AIDS virus will have for treating or preventing the disease. He said anti-viral drugs developed to kill HIV-1 may also work against HIV-2, and vaccine

Dallas Morning News (May 7, 1987).

makers may be able to aim their efforts at parts of the two viruses that are identical.

HIV-2 is genetically similar to SIV, which causes an AIDS-like disease in monkeys.

The Dallas Morning News (May 7, 1987).

Monkeys and AIDS-Immunization Connection

Dr. Eva Lee Snead, M.D., of San Antonio, has come upon evidence that there is a link between AIDS and immunizations. The polio vaccine, begun about 30 years ago, was administered to millions of people, now in their late 30's, and was sent to 3rd world countries throughout the globe and given to millions of Africans, Haitians, Brazilians, and others.

Simian Virus 40, Polio Vaccines and AIDS

The AIDS virus is now called HIV. According to Dr. Snead, researchers conclude that it is not a newcomer, but much like SV-40 (Simian Virus 40), suspected of being carried by the African green monkey (simians). *SV-40 causes a clinical syndrome indistinguishable from AIDS.* It also causes birth defects, leukemias, and other forms of malignancy.

Most people would be repulsed at the thought of green monkey soup. But what if it was stained pink and put on a sugar cube?

Dr. Snead went to the medical library to get more information about the African green monkey and Simian Virus 40 (SV-40), and learned far more than anticipated. She noted that strangely all reference to SV-40 abruptly stopped in 1964.

Suddenly her eyes fell upon the phrase, "Execretion [sic] of SV-40 after oral administration of contaminated polio

Voice of Liberty (Fall 1987).

vaccine."

"Of course," she thought, "practically the whole world has received this immunization." She felt she had solved the riddle not only of AIDS, but also of the dramatic increase in cases of childhood leukemia, birth defects, other malignancies and many chronic, degenerative conditions.

AIDS is a virus. A virus is now described as any particle, natural or man-made, which can enter a cell and cause this cell to make copies of itself. The power of reproduction exists only in the living cell. SV-40 has the ability of carry-information "piggyback" into a cell, and may have that type of role in AIDS. SV-40 hybridizes with other viruses. It may predispose to secondary viral infection by destroying the immune system. SV-40 was present, yet passed unde-tected, in the early stages of Salk and Sabine polio vaccine.

M. Pawlitta describes a new "papovavirus" (the family to which SV-40 belongs). It is called Lymphotropic Papovavirus (LPV). Reportedly it was isolated in 1979 from a culture derived from an African green monkey lymph node.

SV-40, AIDS Symptoms Same

If SV-40 caused the development of AIDS and other dis-eases, it would cause symptoms of the disease in experimental situations:

Interference of T-Cell Formation. The green monkey cell cultures inhibit proliferation of thymocites (T-cells — thymus-immune system). This can be caused by direct inoc-ulation or by contact with individuals who harbor the virus. Such individuals may have received immunizations, or be one of the countless technicians who handled the monkeys or the monkey cells.

Development of Malignancies. When SV-40 is introduced

Voice of Liberty (Fall 1987).

into experimental animals it causes large percentages of them to develop malignancies. Arthur J. Snider wrote, "There was some evidence the SV-40 virus ... when put in human tissue, could cause some cell changes suggestive of tumor growth."

Body Wasting. SV-40 causes decrease in protein production (all cells, tissues, bones, and all solid parts of the body are made of protein. Ed.). Experiments with hamsters showed decrease of albumen, indicative of severe body wasting.

Increased Birth Defects, Tumors, Leukemias. Results indicate high frequency of leukemia and human mongolism. Mongoloid children are also reported to show an increase in incidence of leukemia.

J. J. Mulvhill, M.D., reports a close association of some birth defects with malignancies, especially leukemias, neurological defects, and vascular tumors. "Any further descriptions of such associations exhibit features strongly *reminiscent to the syndrome described as "AIDS" in the gay community.* Immunodeficiency is constantly associated with them, including development of unusual pneumonias, parasitic conditions, vasculitis, leukemias, etc."

Reportedly Dr. Snead obtained much of her material from FDA through Freedom of Information Act, going back 30 years, showing that FDA has known this information for years! In 1960 World Health Organization issued a bulletin informing about undesirable viruses that might be encountered in vaccines. In 1961 the live virus was started and presumed safe. In 1963 *Science Digest*, Journal of New York Academy of Science, reported that humans are susceptible to simian tumor virus. *Science Digest* spoke of he "near disaster" of the polio immunization program.

February 1977 *Atlantic Monthly* reported the contamination of millions of Americans with SV-40. In 1977 the first case of officially acknowledged diagnosed acquired immunodeficiency was reported in a Northern European female M.D. in Africa. Many such reports were to follow. The disease is now called AIDS.

Why are FDA and CDC not telling the public these matters? So long as CDC is given millions of dollars to conduct phoney research, they are going to deny that the cause of AIDS might have already been discovered! (Editor).

The Voice of Liberty (Decatur, Georgia, Fall 1987).

Horses Too — Similar Viruses in Other Animals Besides Monkeys

Veterinarian Studies Similarities Between Equine Virus and AIDS

PULLMAN, WASH. — The study of Equine Infectious Anemia (EIA) may play a role in finding a way to control the AIDS virus, according to a Washington State University veterinary professor ....

EIA and AIDS belong to the same group of viruses, the lentiviruses, according to McGuire. As a result, both are similar in how they infect the host.

Researchers at the university are studying how the immune system in a horse responds to the virus once it enters cells in the body and ways to prevent the virus from entering the cells.

McGuire says it's still too early to say what his research will uncover.

Although EIA viruses are not fatal they do cause cyclic periods of illness. Infected horses develop fevers and start to lose red blood cells, becoming anemic.

If they successfully fight off the virus with their natural

Doctor of Veterinary Medicine (August 1987).

immune system they become reasonably healthy again, McGuire says. But through a mutation-like change of the virus' genetic makeup, a variation of the original virus makes the horse ill again, until its immune system again counters it.

Eventually, something in the horse's immune system recognizes that the variations of the virus are all the same in some respect and the cyclic periods of illness end. At that point the horse becomes a "silent carrier" of the virus.

If the horse survives all of that, it is either relegated to a life of being quarantined or it is destroyed.

Depending on state regulations, EIA-infected horses cannot be transported from state to state or across international borders, according to McGuire. And infected show horses cannot be taken to shows.

Doctor of Veterinary Medicine (August 1987). Used by permission.

What About Sheep!

AIDS Research in Sheep Generates New Concerns; Colorado Scientists Fear Untold Human Impact

FORT COLLINS, COLO. — Colorado State University research on an AIDS-like virus in sheep raises the suspicion that the human AIDS virus may be even more lethal than generally believed.

The research found that a lentivirus in sheep, used as a model for the human AIDS virus, directly causes lung and brain diseases, arthritis, and mastitis, and inflammation of female mammary glands that provide milk for offspring.

The investigation also provides insight into the possibility that the AIDS virus might be transmitted via mother's milk to children.

Doctor of Veterinary Medicine (October 1987).

As well, the actual virus and not secondary infections, as currently believed, may be the direct cause of AIDS-related pneumonia, particularly in children.

Researchers also speculate that the AIDS virus may be linked to anemia in humans because an equine lentivirus that is highly similar to the sheep lentivirus produces that effect in horses.

"These are problems that physicians should be on the lookout for," advises James C. DeMartini, a pathology professor in charge of a team of Colorado State pathologists and microbiologists involved in the ongoing research.

The research indicates people possibly might undergo these problems without initially knowing that they are infected with AIDS.

"These problems are not recognized as classical symptoms of AIDS," DeMartini says. "Our research implies that they can occur without the AIDS disease first being detected in a person."

The sheep lentivirus causes slowly occurring disease. The AIDS virus is a human lentivirus.

The sheep research, which stemmed from the university's substantial effort in the last few years to help Peru increase sheep production, supports new scientific evidence that suggests the AIDS virus directly might cause lung and brain diseases.

Doctor of Veterinary Medicine (October 1987). Used by permission.

Goats?
Similar Viruses in Other Animals Besides Monkeys

A very similar lentivirus is 100 percent lethal to sheep and goats, slowly destroying the brains of the infected animals. It is now postulated and feared that virus infected persons

Dr. Kaldahl, *Special Report: AIDS*

Origin of AIDS

who do not develop AIDS will, over a period of many years, develop a slowly progressive dementia [loss/impairment of mental powers] from the slow death of infected brain cells. Clinical reports of this disturbing event are now beginning to appear in the medical literature.

Dr. Paul E. Kaldahl, Pathologist, *Special Report: AIDS* (Noebel/Lutton/Cameron), p. 33.

From Monkeys to Men Who Practiced Monkey Business

From where has this horror come? Many researchers and a forum of medical experts interviewed on the NBC News Special Report, LIFE, DEATH AND AIDS (aired January 21, 1986), believe that the virus mutated from a green monkey virus in Central Africa. Some tribal rituals mingle human and animal blood, and so the virus is thought to have entered Central Africans' bloodstreams, traveled by Central Africans to Haiti, from Haitian male prostitutes to vacationing homosexual men from New York City, and from them to bisexual men, intravenous drug abusers, and the heterosexual population.

NFD Journal (October 1987).

Original Carrier of AIDS Averaged 250 Men Per Year

A California journalist has identified for the first time the person he calls the "Typhoid Mary" of the AIDS epidemic — a Canadian airline steward whom medical researchers have implicated in the initial spread of the deadly disease in North America.

Randy Shilts, in a book recently published, said he uncovered the identity of the man whom researchers for the national Centers for Disease Control in Atlanta referred to only as "Patient Zero" when compiling information about

Shilts, *And the Band Played On* (1987).

the disease in the early 1980s.

Shilts identified the man as Gaetan Dugas of Montreal, who may have contracted the disease through sexual contact with Africans in Europe, and then spread the infection through sexual contact with American men beginning in the late 1970s.

According to Shilts, Dugas took a leave of absence from his job as a steward after he became ill in 1980 and traveled around the continent using free airline passes. Shilts said Dugas' good looks and French-Canadian accent made him popular with homosexual men, but that popularity left a deadly trail. Shilts says that at least 40 of the first 248 homosexual men diagnosed with the illness in the United States had had sex with Dugas or with someone who had.

In the book, *And the Band Played On: Policy, People and the AIDS Epidemic*, Shilts said Dugas, who was diagnosed with AIDS in 1980 at the age of 28, had sexual relations with an average of 250 men per year even after he became ill.

Rethink Nonjudgmental Stand

Many years ago, homosexuality was considered a sin. Over the last several decades, modern physicians redefined it as a disease. Just a few years ago, modern medicine, led by the psychiatrists, removed homosexuality from the lexicon of diseases, calling it an alternative life-style. (The implication of the word "alternative" is that one is just as good as the other.) By removing the traditional social taboos against homosexual behavior, doctors weakened the traditional barriers of fear and guilt that had long served, at least partially, to reduce the incidence of blatant homosexual behavior. When in American history have homosexuals

Dr. Mendelsohn, *Special Report: AIDS* (September 30, 1985).

found it so easy to have the contact with multiple partners that appears to be a prime predisposing factor in AIDS? It makes little difference whether the mechanism of AIDS causation is traumatic, bacterial, viral, or immunologic; a major determinant still remains the number of sexual partners.

Because of AIDS, doctors should begin to rethink their nonjudgmental stand on certain homosexual behavior patterns. Perhaps the common denominator of both these modern epidemics — AIDS and herpes — is promiscuity. Maybe the first step doctors can take in an effort to discourage relations with multiple sexual partners and the diseases that such behavior leads to is to abandon the euphemism "sexually active" and to call promiscuity by its real name.

Dr. Robert Mendelsohn, *Special Report: AIDS* (Noebel/Cameron/Lutton, September 30, 1985).

If we do not stop homosexual conduct, we will not stop the spread of AIDS.

Dr. Fred Schwarz, M.D., *Newsletter* (November 15, 1985).

Gays to Blame

AIDS Takes Many Lives
But Claims Few Victims

WASHINGTON — On and on it goes, the campaign to prove that AIDS "is everybody's disease." It isn't very convincing.

People magazine does a cover story on AIDS victims. The victim on the cover is a 15-year-old hemophiliac. It's touching but not exactly typical.

The next volley comes from *Newsweek*. This is a particu-

Sobran, Kilpatrick, *Universal Press Syndicate* (1987).

larly transparent effort. The cover shows 24 AIDS victims, of both sexes and various ages and races, to suggest that the disease is now reaching a representative cross section of the population.

INSIDE ARE 12 pages of photos, laid out as in a high school yearbook, of "302 men, women, and children struck down by the epidemic in the 12 months ending last week. They range in age from an infant of one to a widow of 87, and they come from every walk of life from mailman to banker, from housewife to superstar."

The text keeps pounding the theme. It admits that 90 percent of those who get AIDS are homosexuals and junkies. "But," it stresses, "there are doctors here and lawyers, bankers and brokers, scholars and preachers, athletes and war heroes, a member of Congress and a bishop of the church."

Look closer. These are all largely male occupations. Nobody ever said that all homosexuals are hairdressers and interior decorators. Besides, most people who get AIDS don't get it at the office.

Of the 24 people shown on the cover, six are women. Of the 302 shown inside, only a dozen are women. The great majority are young men, and 40 of them are from San Francisco. Some cross section.

AIDS ISN'T essentially a homosexual or venereal disease. It's a disease anyone can get. It merely owes the number of its current victims, the large majority of whom are male homosexuals, to male homosexuality. In that respect, it's like hepatitis, a disease that also has an especially high frequency among homosexual men.

The propaganda organs of the "new morality," *Newsweek* prominent among them, are using AIDS, perversely enough, not to warn against homosexuality but to

Sobran, Kilpatrick, *Universal Press Syndicate* (1987).

legitimize it. This accounts for the oddly elusive quality of the public discussion of AIDS. On the one hand, we are asked to review AIDS as the latest form of homosexual victimization, a tragic new chapter in the lachrymose history of a persecuted people. On the other hand, we are to be cautioned that AIDS is likely to strike anyone, even the banker next door.

Since even the experts are sometimes longer on advocacy than on hard knowledge, it's best to refer the issue to common sense. The two or three known AIDS viruses have presumably existed, probably in obscure parts of Africa, since time immemorial. New life forms don't spring into existence very often.

Most diseases show up fairly soon after they are caught and can be coped with by modern medical treatment. AIDS is new to us, if not to nature. It remains dormant for years. Thousands of people had it before anyone had become aware of it. Having gotten the jump on detection, it now defies cures.

It resembles hepatitis, again, in being circulated with special velocity by certain practices that most people consider unsavory and unsanitary. We don't usually think of male homosexuals and intravenous drug users as "victims" of hepatitis; we think of them as courting it.

We have known about hepatitis and other diseases, including venereal diseases, for a long time now. Those who turned out to be spreading AIDS have also been spreading other things. Their behavior is obviously risky and reckless. It shouldn't amaze us that they have given speedy circulation to other disorders that, but for them, would have remained rare or unheard of. There is no reason to assume that AIDS will be the last pathological innovation of the new sex-and-drugs network created by the "new morality" in

Sobran, Kilpatrick, *Universal Press Syndicate* (1987).

conjunction with modern mobility.

The 15-year-old hemophiliac who depends on other people's bodily fluids is truly a "victim" of AIDS. Those whose behavior gave it to him belong in a more ambiguous category. By all means they should be cured, if possible. The rest of us, though, should be spared all this piteous attitudinizing over their plight.

Charts Don't Lie

The following statistics should silence the myth makers. AIDS is a homosexual disease transmitted to females mainly via bisexual males or drugs.

AIDS WEEKLY SURVEILLANCE REPORT — UNITED STATES
AIDS PROGRAM, CENTER FOR INFECTIOUS DISEASES
CENTERS FOR DISEASE CONTROL

UNITED STATES CASES REPORTED TO CDC **JUNE 22, 1987**

A. TRANSMISSION CATEGORIES	MALES				FEMALES				TOTAL			
	Since Jan. 1		Cumulative		Since Jan. 1		Cumulative		Since Jan. 1		Cumulative	
ADULTS/ADOLESCENTS	Number	(%)	Number	(%)	Number	(%)	Number	(%)	Number	(%)	Number	(%)
Homosexual/Bisexual Male	5559	(72)	24341	(71)					5559	(67)	24341	(66)
Intravenous (IV) Drug Abuser	906	(12)	4821	(14)	257	(44)	1270	(50)	1163	(14)	6091	(17)
Homosexual Male and IV Drug Abuser	561	(7)	2804	(8)					561	(7)	2804	(8)
Hemophilia/Coagulation Disorder	88	(1)	328	(1)	1	(0)	8	(0)	89	(1)	336	(1)
Heterosexual Cases	120	(2)	683	(2)	173	(30)	736	(29)	293	(4)	1419	(4)
Transfusion, Blood/Components	154	(2)	494	(1)	82	(14)	270	(11)	236	(3)	764	(2)
Undetermined	289	(4)	864	(3)	65	(11)	251	(10)	354	(4)	1115	(3)
SUBTOTAL [% of all cases]	7677	[93]	34335	[93]	578	[7]	2535	[7]	8255	[100]	36870	[100]
CHILDREN												
Hemophilia/Coagulation Disorder	6	(11)	27	(10)			2	(1)	6	(6)	29	(6)
Parent with/at risk of AIDS	40	(70)	203	(72)	41	(82)	200	(85)	81	(76)	403	(78)
Transfusion, Blood/Components	6	(11)	39	(14)	3	(6)	22	(9)	9	(8)	61	(12)
Undetermined	5	(9)	12	(4)	6	(12)	11	(5)	11	(10)	23	(4)
SUB TOTAL [% of all cases]	57	[53]	281	[54]	50	[47]	235	[46]	107	[100]	516	[100]
TOTAL [% of all cases]	7734	[92]	34616	[93]	628	[8]	2770	[7]	8362	[100]	37386	[100]

AIDS Weekly Surveillance Report, United States AIDS Program, Center for Infectious Diseases, Centers for Disease Control (June 22, 1987).

The Big AIDS Con Job

We are loudly informed, officially, that the nation's blood-bank supplies are safer than ever. Meanwhile, some physicians are advising patients contemplating elective surgery to build up a supply of their own blood for transfusion. Since 1981, 414 Americans have developed fatal cases of AIDS after receiving contaminated blood transfusions, and up to seven hundred more in New York alone may have been fatally infected. Yeah, the nation's blood banks are safer than ever. Dengue fever is down.

We are loudly informed, officially, that AIDS can be contracted only through "exchange of bodily fluids," through "intimate sexual contact." Great. But the virus has turned up in saliva and in tears, and the actors' unions have negotiated an end to big kissing scenes on tube and screen. Nevertheless, in many parts of the country AIDS patients are acquiring a legal right to access to workplace and classroom. By the year 1990, absent a cure, some 250,000 Americans are expected to die of AIDS.

Now comes *Newsweek* with what in many respects is a brilliant piece on AIDS, focused on a heroic doctor in the Bronx named Gerald Friedland who is in the front lines of AIDS treatment. There's a funny thing about the article, however. With one exception — a gay male named Robert — all of the AIDS patients described in any detail are heterosexual, with a needle usually in the background. The ratio is about a dozen heterosexuals to one gay. *Newsweek* apparently intended to convey the impression that this ratio represents reality.

What appears to be going on is a great coverup, cleanup. *Newsweek* is industriously trying to put distance between AIDS and homosexuality, whatever the facts in the matter.

National Review (August 15, 1986).

Origin of AIDS

AIDS is being accorded victim status, as if it were analogous to racial discrimination rather than a public-health problem. The unknowns about the transmission of the disease are, to say the least, not being stressed.

Newsweek and the rest of the culture appear to be engaging in a sort of homosexual-protection operation, shielding gay sex from connection with the epidemic. Why? Everyone knows the facts.

National Review (August 15, 1986).

Scared to Die

... a 28-year-old patient says, "I'm very scared to die such a young man. I'd like a little more time."

The man is not gay. He is married and the father of two children. But he readily admits to a life of promiscuity and a history of many liaisons with prostitutes.

Gerald Clarke, *Time:* "AIDS: A Growing Threat" (August 12, 1985). Copyright 1985 *Time Inc.* All rights reserved. Reprinted by permission from *Time.*

Prostitutes' AIDS Risk High

ATLANTA (AP) — Early results from a study indicate that drug use is rampant among street prostitutes and as many as half are infected with the virus that causes AIDS.

Researchers from Howard University, who are surveying as many as 200 prostitutes, found that 13 out of the first 26 they tested were infected with AIDS virus. The findings were presented Monday in Atlanta at the annual convention of the American Society for Microbiology. [A]ll 13, as well as nine of the 13 who weren't infected, were users of injectible drugs, which would place them at risk for AIDS regardless of their sexual habits. The disease is transmitted most often through sexual contact or contaminated drug needles.

The Evansville Courier (March 3, 1987).

Hookers Hook Victims

Dr. William Hazeltine [sic] of Harvard's Dana-Farber Cancer Institute has reported the following in Congressional testimony regarding the potential for AIDS spread through female prostitutes:

"... There is accumulating evidence that infection is transmitted from prostitutes to their customers. A recent

Dr. Hazeltine [sic]

Prostitutes

study conducted by the United States Army revealed that five percent of the United States soldiers reporting to venereal disease clinics in Berlin are now infected with the AIDS virus ..."

Dr. William Hazeltine [sic]

Hookers and Russian Roulette

One of the major routes of AIDS transmission in Africa appears to be prostitutes. Although prostitution may not be any more rampant in Central Africa than in New York City, it exists very openly there, driven by poverty and the lack of other work for young African women.

A study by a team of 12 scientists and researchers examining the spread of AIDS in East Africa found low-income prostitutes in Kenya averaged 963 partners a year, middle-income ones 124 annually. The latter's customers are frequently foreign tourists and international businessmen who will carry the AIDS virus back to Europe and America. One American AIDS expert says African prostitutes have such high HIV-infection rates that their clients would have "better odds playing Russian roulette."

Within Africa, transmission of AIDS is also facilitated by a high tolerance for extramarital affairs by men, as well as wide acceptance for unmarried men and women having many sexual partners. This promiscuous life-style is reflected in studies showing higher incidence of sexually transmitted diseases among Africans than among Westerners.

Readers Digest (June 1987).

Howard University tested 26 street prostitutes and found that half of them were carrying the AIDS virus — figures even more worrisome than a Miami survey showing that 40 percent of hookers carrying the AIDS virus.

Carl T. Rowan, *Washington UPI.*

Fear of AIDS Chills Sex Industry

"Pleasure Palaces" in Nevada and Japan Stress Tests, Preventive Measures as They Try to Lure Customers

The world's oldest profession is in a slump. Reason: The world's newest plague — AIDS.

Take Nevada. Legal prostitution has flourished in the state since the 1860s, weathering even the worst of times with barely a ripple. But health officials say patronage of such coyly named bordellos as the Chicken Ranch, Desert Doll House, and Mustang Ranch has been off by as much as 40 percent.

The panic over what remains mostly a U.S. phenomenon has even reached Tokyo's notorious Yoshiwara red-light district, where all that whistles nowadays is a frigid winter wind. "I've been here 40 years," complained one Tokyo *mama-san* as she sourly surveyed a desolate club, "and business has never been worse." The drop for some establishments is estimated at 90 percent — a decline accelerated by the widely publicized AIDS death of a Kobe prostitute.

On both sides of the Pacific, the industry is struggling to rally. Yokohama's massage parlors, frequented by American servicemen, prominently display signs pledging that women are *"eizu"* free. A hundred Yoshiwara hostesses voluntarily took blood tests for exposure to the AIDS virus. One Nevada prostitute even claims she submits to weekly AIDS tests rather than the monthly check demanded by law. "We're at more risk than the men," laments a 27-year-old blonde, whose hospital-clean cubicle smacks more of a sorority house than a place where sex is for hire. Many

Chaze, Hawkins, *U.S. News & World Report* (February 16, 1987).

Prostitutes

brothel owners require customers to use prophylactics. "Condoms available on request at no extra charge," reads a sign at the Sagebrush Ranch near Carson City.

Safe So Far

Nevada, the only part of America where prostitution is legal, began requiring AIDS screening in mid-1986. While none of the 350 women checked by the state has flunked the test, eight others seeking work as prostitutes have been turned away as infected. Authorities claim no one has gotten AIDS in any of Nevada's 37 brothels. But many hundreds of unregistered prostitutes work illegally, and no one knows if the screening has become common practice among them. The assumption is that it has not.

A bellhop at Reno's Hilton Hotel says that many guests still ask directions to the nearest brothel. "But when we remind them about AIDS," he says, "they stop being caught up in the idea of legalized prostitution." Robert Nellis, senior health advisor with the Nevada Division of Health, maintains that a "john" stands a much better chance of getting AIDS from a free-lancer: "It's probably safer to go ... to a brothel than pick up a prostitute on the street or in one of the casinos when you don't know if they've ever been checked. But we're guaranteeing nothing. It's always a possibility someone could get it [AIDS] in between checkups."

The Japanese alarm over AIDS has spread far beyond what the numbers — 26 cases nationwide, with 18 deaths — might seem to justify. But to the Japanese, physically isolated and tending to view themselves as unique, the disease always seemed another's nightmare. The death of the AIDS-afflicted 29-year-old Kobe prostitute changed that.

Whipped into a near frenzy by lurid, full-color specials in the mass media showing symptoms and victims — "Do you

Chaze, Hawkins, *U.S. News & World Report* (February 16, 1987).

have AIDS lurking in your body?'' queried one magazine —
anxious callers flooded Tokyo's new 24-hour AIDS hot line
with 247,000 calls during its first week. Many were from
wives worried about wayward husbands.

White Peril?

Increasingly, the scare carries xenophobic overtones.
Hot-line callers fret that the foreigner with whom they had a
fling will prove to be an AIDS carrier. Massage parlors and
even legitimate public baths have taken to posting "No For-
eigners" signs. In Kanegawa prefecture, host to 19
American military installations, officials want all Seventh
Fleet sailors tested. The Health and Welfare Ministry is
reported to be weighing a new policy denying entry to for-
eigners suspected as AIDS carriers.

For the present, the Japanese are taking precautions by
boycotting their celebrated pleasure quarters as never
before. In garish Yoshiwara, tuxedo-clad barkers still man
the doors of dozens of girlie clubs. But the streets, filled
with hard-drinking businessmen and tourists only a year
ago, today are empty, and the barkers' professional cheer
has given way to a forlorn weariness. Time drags by in
grumpy silence. "How's business?" grimaces one barker to
a passer-by's question. "Lousy."

William L. Chaze with Steve L. Hawkins, *U.S News & World Report*
(Copyright February 16, 1987). Used by permission.

Quarantine

(Check section on Testing also.)

Syphilis Never Had Civil Rights. Why Does AIDS?

There is a sexually transmitted disease with a very long incubation period, that is life threatening, and incurable. AIDS? No, syphilis prior to 1945. It was defeated by routing epidemiologic techniques. Everyone was tested when hospitalized, married, or inducted into the armed forces until the affected were identified, counseled, and all contacts followed.

Prior to this public health effort, syphilis filled one-half of the hospital beds in the United States, just as AIDS will do in five years unless the federal government changes its lackadaisical attitude.

Syphilis never had civil rights. Why is AIDS different? What about the rights of health care workers who frequently are not informed of those with AIDS-related complex and AIDS, but are required to work with infected body fluids without giving informed consent? I feel the legal profession will have a field day when a health care worker and his family come down with AIDS and nobody warned them.

Dr. Olav II. Alvig, *American Medical News* (December 20, 1985).

Gay-Baiting Crackpots

Newsweek, September 23, 1985, wrote, "For the first time, talk of a quarantine, previously confined to a handful of gay-baiting crackpots, has begun appearing in such high-minded forums as the *Washington Post* — while William Curran, professor of legal medicine at Harvard Medical School, told *Newsweek* that he is preparing standby regulations for cities to apply in confining AIDS patients who

Newsweek (September 23, 1985) and *Washington Post* (September 8, 1985).

willfully persist in giving the disease to others.''

Dr. Richard Restak was quoted in the *Washington Post* for September 8, 1985, as saying, "Quarantines have been very effective in beating outbreaks of scarlet fever, smallpox, and typhoid in this century. Indeed, by protecting the well from the ill we follow a long-established, sensible, and ultimately compassionate course. Throughout history true humanitarianism has traditionally involved the compassionate but firm segregation of those afflicted with communicable diseases from the well. By carrying out such a policy, diseases have been contained."

Newsweek (September 23, 1985) and *Washington Post* (September 8, 1985).

A Plague

Dr. James Curran stated, "This is a plague and a menace, and I see nothing wrong with quarantine on a constitutional level."

J. Adler/N. F. Greenberg/M. Hager/P. McKillop/T. Namuth, *Newsweek*: "The AIDS Conflict" (September 23, 1985).

A Lethal Virus

We then would have to use public health measures including quarantine, to stop those people who deliberately infect another individual by sharing an infected needle or by having sexual intercourse when they know they themselves are infected, thus deliberately (spreading) this potentially lethal virus to another person.

Dr. Vernon A. Mark, Associate Professor of Surgery, Harvard Medical School, Interview with Dr. Ed Rowe, President, New National AIDS Prevention Institute (March 1987).

What Answers for AIDS?

Would you send your child to school with a kid who has AIDS? Do you want potential AIDS victims screened

Gergen, *U.S. News & World Report* (September 23, 1985).

before they come to work with you? Or what would you do if you discovered your dental hygienist had the disease?

Such questions, once considered remote, are now confronting millions of Americans worried that a new plague may be striking our society.

American doctors first identified AIDS victims only four years ago, and there was only a small number of cases, mostly confined to the homosexual community. Today, there are more than 13,000 known victims, the number is doubling every year and the disease is reaching into the heterosexual community. Unlike bubonic plague and tuberculosis of earlier times, AIDS also seems to kill everyone it infects.

A deep fear now grips many neighborhoods, and it, too, is spreading. A national poll earlier this month found that AIDS had become the second most dreaded illness, second only to cancer but ahead of heart disease. New York City parents angrily boycotted schools this fall when authorities admitted a single, unidentified child. School officials in Florida, Indiana, and California have excluded AIDS victims from public classrooms. The U.S. military is also beginning to screen recruits for evidence of exposure to this disease.

The fear of AIDS has reached a point where a national response is needed. Health and Human Services Secretary Margaret Heckler has declared AIDS the No. 1 public-health problem ....

Now, Mrs. Heckler, acting in concert with the President, needs to assemble the best health authorities in the country to assure we are on a proper policy course and draft guide lines that can help parents, school officials, employers, and others trying to sort out difficult questions. The country needs not only more information but also a greater sense of

Gergen, *U.S. News & World Report* (September 23, 1985).

security. Too many people are on the verge of hysteria.

At the heart of the matter is the necessity that, as we await yet another breakthrough in medicine, we treat both the sick and the well with fairness and compassion.

Those who have acquired the disease deserve dignity and care. Although homosexuality may be abhorrent to many Americans, fear of this disease should not drive us to abandon our commitment to fair-minded treatment of all citizens.

But there are limits to what should be expected of society, too. Those who are well have a right to live reasonably free from fear and contamination from this disease. They should not be compelled to take unnecessary risks, especially with their children ....

In such circumstances, we should pay heed to Dr. Richard Restak, a neurologist and author of *The Brain*. In a recent article in the *Washington Post* that has stirred controversy in the nation's capital, Dr. Restak argued that until we know more, the "truly humanitarian position" is to consider forms of quarantine for victims of AIDS.

"Quarantines have been very effective in beating outbreaks of scarlet fever, smallpox and typhoid in this century. Indeed, by protecting the well from the ill, we follow long-established, sensible, and ultimately compassionate course .... By carrying out such a policy, diseases have been contained."

Throughout our history, Americans have struggled — usually with success — to strike a proper balance between the rights of the individual and those of society. We must find that balance once again today.

David R. Gergen, *U.S. News & World Report* (Copyright September 23, 1985). Used by permission.

Fears Aren't False; Rights Must Be Limited

INDIANAPOLIS — Is it persecution of a minority to demand that public officials protect innocent citizens against a killer disease, AIDS?

Does a quarantine of AIDS carriers abuse their civil rights and rape the Constitution?

No, it is not persecution. It is common sense. Even Dr. James Curran, a Harvard health official, has said: "This is a plague. I see nothing wrong with quarantine."

Protection of the innocent is the basic responsibility of government, but they are not being protected. AIDS has been contracted by children from blood transfusions, babies from mothers' milk, women from artificial insemination, lab workers from infected blood.

We are told not to worry about casual contact, yet the nurses who cared for Rock Hudson in Paris burned their garments after each shift and fed him off paper plates with plastic table service.

We are told casual contact with carriers is "believed safe," but *no one* can guarantee *anything*. *New York* magazine reported mosquitoes might carry the virus; *USA Today* reported preliminary findings from a study in Africa showed it might be spread by casual household contact.

Yet we are accused of being fearmongers, haters, and abusers of civil rights by demanding that public officials bend over backward toward protecting the public rather than permit a handful of infected children into a classroom.

The Indianapolis Star reported specialists saying "it is virtually impossible to catch the disease from mosquito bites or ordinary day-to-day activity such as shaking hands." Note "virtually." Sincere "experts" always qualify their statements with ambiguities — "virtually," "usually," "most of

Boys, *USA Today* (November 4, 1985).

the time." It's like saying the acrobat "virtually" caught the trapeze — but really fell and broke his sincere neck!

Experts give me no assurance at all. Sure I'm concerned about the innocent carriers of AIDS, but since we don't *know* the facts, we should err in favor of caution.

Seven percent of AIDS carriers don't know how they contracted the disease; it's what we *don't* know about AIDS that may end up killing us. Responsible people will assume the worst until experts can speak authoritatively.

Sodomy is an evil that may be the catalyst for a devastating plague that may make us look back longingly for the days of TB, typhoid, diphtheria, and polio. TB was the chief cause of death in the USA until 1909 and was 11th as late as 1954. It was illegal not to report diseased persons to health officials; whole communities were X-rayed to identify and treat carriers. Why should AIDS carriers be treated differently?

Public officials must not be intimidated by the clenched fist of the militant homosexual or his bedfellows, the sanctimonious liberals. Officials must act against AIDS even if innocent people might be hurt. While not desirable, it is preferable to a repeat of the Black Death of the 1300s that prompted Froissart's casual words: "A third of the world died."

Don Boys, *USA Today* (November 4, 1985).

He Suspected the Cook

Typhoid Mary, [a] blond, blue-eyed, square-jawed cook worked in homes and institutions in New York between 1897 and 1910. In 1906, when 23,000 people were dying of typhoid, the cook, named Mary Mallon, went to work for a wealthy banker in Oyster Bay, N.Y. Almost immediately six members of the household came down with typhoid. When

The Detroit News

no other households reported cases, investigators were summoned.

After eliminating other causes — the milk, the water supply, the drainage, a single inside toilet — an investigator began looking for a human carrier and focused on the cook, who had left the banker's kitchen and moved to Tuxedo, N.Y., where there were fresh cases of typhoid.

Checking back, the engineer found that almost everywhere Mary Mallon had worked, there was typhoid. She was an innocent victim of her own body chemistry and, by failing to wash her hands after going to the restroom, she was contaminating the food she prepared. The investigator confronted Mary with his evidence and asked for specimens of her body wastes. She refused to cooperate and, out of fear for her safety and freedom, fled. It later took five policemen to subdue her.

Though confined for four years in a hospital, Mary Mallon never cooperated with public health officials, who offered to remove her gall bladder and render her harmless. When released, she went back to work as a cook — at a hospital, where typhoid broke out immediately. "Typhoid Mary" was again arrested and confined for the rest of her life.

The Detroit News

Florida Proposes AIDS Lockup Wards

Florida is proposing special lockup wards for AIDS carriers who appear to be knowingly spreading the disease and others who refuse to submit to AIDS testing.

The draft policy paper by the Department of Health and Rehabilitative Services in Tallahassee is primarily aimed at prostitutes and others who knowingly expose others to the deadly virus, Health Secretary Gregory Coler said.

Detroit News (January 27, 1988).

Quarantine

Judges would determine when adult AIDS patients pose a threat to others, either through having sex without a condom or through the sharing of needles. Those accused [w]ould have the right to an attorney, to cross-examine witnesses and submit to testing to disprove the allegation.

Detroit News (January 27, 1988).

What's Wrong With Our Heads?

We are dealing with a virus that certainly is as lethal as smallpox, and possibly much more lethal. Nobody in their right mind would do anything other than restrict the activities of a person with smallpox.

Dr. John Seale, *Special Report: AIDS* (Noebel/Lutton/Cameron).

Quarantines Work

The AIDS virus has no "civil rights." Quarantines have been very effective in beating outbreaks of scarlet fever, smallpox, and typhoid in this century.

Dr. Richard Restak, *Executive Intelligence Review*: "Medical Experts on AIDS Danger" (September 27, 1985).

Rock Hudson's Nurses Burned Their Clothes

The point about AIDS is that there is a whole lot we don't know about it. Tomorrow we will find out something else, beyond the vague business about how AIDS is only known to be communicable through sexual intercourse. (Once? Twice? 100?, the story here is not even clear) and, contaminated needles how else? By no other means? Well, then, how come they acted as they did in Paris? There you may have read (in small print) when Rock Hudson was discharged, all the nurses who attended to him — and this was in a modern hospital, not a witch doctor's hut — were made to burn their dresses. The patient was fed on paper and plastic plates, with plastic forks and spoons — which were destroyed.

Buckley, *National Review* (November 18, 1985).

Quarantine

So what, a non-hysterical mother is entitled to ask herself, is a Paris hospital up to, safeguarding the hygiene of nurses and doctors and hospital employees, that she should not also be up to, safeguarding the hygiene of Suzy and Johnny who are asked to go to school and share meals, and games, and rough and tumble, with someone suffering from AIDS?

William F. Buckley Jr., *National Review* (November 18, 1985).

Schools — AIDS Contagious?

Lice Out — AIDS In

Throughout history, pandemics have not been stopped by "miracle cures," but by the society imposing strict public health measures to stop the contagion from spreading. If the disease is contained, then medical research — if adequately funded — has the time to make research breakthroughs. It is one of the ABCs of public health, that the very first thing that must be done, is to identify those who are carrying the deadly disease and isolate them from healthy people. By this criterion alone, the position so far taken by the CDC in Atlanta and by the government health authorities is incompetent, dangerous, and a violation of every basic precept of public health. In New York City, for example, the law prescribes that children found infested with lice must be sent home from school; but children with AIDS are supposed to stay.

W. J. Hamerman/J. Grauerholz, M.D., FCAP/J. Tennenbaum, Ph.D./ D. Freeman, Ph.D./W. Lillge, M.D./N. Rosinsky, M.D./E. Shapiro, M.D./M. Budman/R. Pauls, M.D., *Executive Intelligence Review*: "Why Is Atlanta CDC Covering Up the AIDS Story" (September 27, 1985), Vol. 12 No. 38.

Schools — AIDS Is Communicable

A Communicable Seven-year-old With AIDS

Dr. Donald Rosenblatt, an internist at Flushing General Hospital, who has treated 100 AIDS victims, testified before Judge Harold Hyman in the Queens, New York school case. Rosenblatt has worked with AIDS cases at Memorial Sloan-Kettering Hospital. From the court transcript:

Dr. Rosenblatt, Flushing General Hospital.

Schools

Dr. Rosenblatt: "It is my opinion that a 7-year-old with AIDS is communicable ... I would say that it is medically unsound for the child to attend classes."

Q. If a student, the AIDS student, throws up, or gets cut or gets in a fight or cries or has a bloody nose, should caution be used?

Dr. Rosenblatt: "Absolutely."

Q. If two children mix cuts ... and one has AIDS, is there any guarantee that the child, the other child, will get AIDS?

Dr. Rosenblatt: "He's in serious trouble."

Dr. Ronald Rosenblatt, Flushing General Hospital

Scratching, Biting, and Spitting

Any grade-school teacher can attest that "body-fluid contamination" in the form of scratching, throwing up, diarrhea, biting, and spitting are everyday fare within a normal schoolroom ....

At this point live AIDS virus has been isolated from blood, semen, serum, saliva, urine, and now tears. If the virus exists in these fluids, the better part of wisdom dictates that we assume the possibility that it can also be transmitted by these routes.

Dr. Richard Restak, *Special Report: AIDS*: (*Washington Post,* Noebel/Lutton/Cameron, September 8, 1985), p. C-4.

It's Hardly Hysteria To Fear This Plague

INDIANAPOLIS — A frigid wind of fear is blowing across the USA, building in intensity over the specter of AIDS. Some suggest this *fear* may be worse then the *fact* — another fairy story from Sodom-by-the-Bay.

Other plagues that hammered this world one after another were not 100 percent deadly. AIDS is. A diagnosis of AIDS is a death sentence. Yet we are told not to be fearful!

Boys, *USA Today* (December 13, 1987).

Homosexuals are trying to sell us a gold brick — that AIDS is not a "gay" disease. When they make up only 2 percent of the population and constitute 75 percent of AIDS carriers, *that* makes it a gay disease.

Homosexual groups promote "safe sex" — the use of condoms and cleanliness before and after acts of perversion. They also suggest men reduce the number of sex partners. Why not total abstinence or observance of normalcy?

They tell us they only "love a little differently." But how can anyone suggest that sodomy is normal, loving, noble, and desirable when it could lead to the death of a friend — or the depletion of the human race?

The more AIDS "jumps the tracks," affecting and infecting normal people, the greater will be the revulsion and fear. Some of us think fear is a normal reaction, especially until all the facts are in.

Politicians who don't have enough guts to make one good sausage link are afraid to antagonize the militant sodomite organizations. Even if it is eventually proved that one cannot contract AIDS by casual contact, don't we have a right to expect our lawmakers to assume the worst when passing relevant laws?

I would not permit my children to go to school where mumps, measles, or meningitis are present, so I sure wouldn't permit them to attend where AIDS is present.

This does not mean I would countenance mistreatment of AIDS victims, especially an innocent (non-sexual) victim. AIDS victims should not be abandoned by family and friends. However, caution should be exercised as with any infectious disease.

The fact is the "experts" don't *know* that AIDS can't be contracted from sneezing, coughing, saliva, or mosquitoes.

Boys, *USA Today* (December 13, 1987).

Schools

And I consider grandstanding "experts" to be irresponsible at best and quacks at worst.

Liberals accuse me of being unfair and outrageous because of my sane and sensible approach about AIDS and its victims. A liberal accusing a ... conservative of being unfair and outrageous is like a skunk accusing a rabbit of having bad breath. Those who are cavalier with innocent lives, who tell us that all we have to fear is fear itself are the unfair and outrageous ones.

Don Boys, president of Associated Christian Schools Curriculum and former Member of Indiana House, *USA Today* (December 13, 1987). Used by permission.

1 in 61 New York City Infants Has AIDS Antibodies, Study Says

NEW YORK — One in every 61 babies born in New York City tested positive for antibodies to the AIDS virus in a month-long study that looked at blood from every infant born in New York state.

State health officials, who provided details of the study Wednesday, said it was all but certain the mothers of 164 infants born in the state and found to be carrying the antibodies were infected with the deadly AIDS virus.

The blood tests performed on 19,157 infants born during a month-long period beginning in late November showed that acquired immune deficiency syndrome (AIDS) has emerged as a leading threat to infant health in New York City. Of about 9,000 babies born in the city during the month, 148 tested positive for AIDS antibodies.

Based on their study, the officials projected that 1,000 babies infected with the AIDS virus will be born in New York State this year, nearly all of them in New York City.

The results provided the first comprehensive look at AIDS infection across the infant and childbearing female

The Detroit News

216

population of an area that includes a high rate of AIDS cases, Health Department spokeswoman Frances Tarlton said.

Reprinted with permission of *The Detroit News*, a Gannett newspaper, copyright 1988.

Koop Wants Campuswide AIDS Test at a University

State College Officials Lukewarm to Idea

LONDON — U.S. Surgeon General C. Everett Koop said Thursday he wants to screen every student at a major American university this spring to study the incidence of AIDS among young adults.

Koop also proposed similar mass AIDS screening at a few high schools in the United States, but said the government had made no decision on either proposal.

Officials at Michigan universities said they support Koop's efforts to learn more about the prevalence of the disease, but predicted completing such a testing program on a college campus would be difficult.

Koop's plan, disclosed at a world meeting on AIDS in London, could prove controversial. Civil libertarians have argued that anonymous screening is an invasion of privacy and that screening of a limited population could be the forerunner of mandatory nationwide testing.

The surgeon general said health officials had yet to choose a university, but it would likely be one in a large city with about 25,000 students.

He said the screening would not be mandatory.

"The goal would be to test everybody in that university in such a way that it's done out in the open, aboveboard. Everyone knows that the blood specimen is not in any way

Glass, *The Detroit News* (January 29, 1988).

tagged," Koop said.

Caesar M. Briefer, director of health services at the University of Michigan, said Koop's idea had some merit as a research project.

"But I also think there are a lot of potential logistical problems in trying to do something like that," said Briefer.

Thomas E. Coyne, vice-president for student services at Western Michigan, agreed.

"First of all, that would have to be voluntary," Coyne said. "I also wonder about what anxiety level would be produced among people on that campus if the report said X percent had AIDS. I would want to move extremely cautiously with an idea of that nature."

Koop said anonymity would be guaranteed and those taking part would have no way of knowing individual results.

The incidence of acquired immune deficiency syndrome is highest among 20- to 24-year-olds, with male homosexuals and drug abusers among those most at risk.

Koop said he also hoped that such screening could be carried out at a few high schools in diverse parts of the country. As examples of the types of places he had in mind, Koop cited Philadelphia or New York's South Bronx in the Northeast and Evansville, Ind., in the Midwest.

Robert Glass (News Staff Writer Robbie Morganfield contributed to this report), *The Detroit News* (Associated Press, January 29, 1988).

The AIDS epidemic has entered the worry stream, the 4-o'clock-in-the-morning concerns. If we do not worry for ourselves, it's for our friends, family, children. Many now routinely pore over scare stories and search for antidotes to anxiety in the progress reports from the medical world.

Nevertheless, it is remarkable how little actual behavior has changed. In the *Atlantic* magazine, Katie Leishman writes, "AIDS may provide the ultimate test of strategies for behavior modification." But she reports on partners of AIDS patients who go on having sex and without condoms, on gay men who cut back but do not cut out unprotected sex, and on people who shield themselves with intuition ....

THERE ARE some who offer a one-word answer to this epidemic: no. Say no to unwed sex. Say no to prostitution. Say no to drugs. But is this to be our sole national-health program: "Say No or Die"? And how do we protect people from those who said yes?

To date 30,000 Americans have been stricken by AIDS, 1,200 of them heterosexuals. We have no idea how many carry the virus. As — not *if* but *as* — AIDS spreads through the population, "no" will become a much more common answer to sex. Testing may become routine, and so will the demand for every kind of protection from education to condoms to clean syringes. But how many more will die before our behavior, public as well as private, is "modified"?

Ellen Goodman, *Detroit News* (February 4, 1987).

Q. Even if I test negative, is it a good idea to be tested every few months?

No. It would be better to change your sexual behavior to minimize risk. A test can only reveal the past, while changing your behavior can influence your future health for the better.

U.S. News & World Report (*Horizons*, April 20, 1987).

Sexual Abstinence

The Blame for AIDS

A movie to be used for AIDS education in York City Schools includes the claim that no one is to blame for AIDS except the virus. I do not question the advisability of using the film, but the notion, recently affirmed by the editor of the *Daily Record*, that no one is responsible except the virus is an example of a dangerous myth that must be challenged.

Underlying this myth is a tendency in our society to disclaim responsibility for individual actions and a false objectivity that prefers to avoid any discussion of morality. Thus when the head of Planned Parenthood came to town, she suggested that the problems resulting from teen-age sexual activity would disappear if Americans would set aside their moral hang-ups and see it as part of normal development.

The myth is that if we can somehow get rid of that old baggage we can put our technical skills to work and solve the problems that face us.

The myth is false because AIDS is spread by dangerous, immoral and irresponsible human actions. It appears to have had its start as an epidemic because of the breakdown of traditional family life and mores in Africa under the pressure of urbanization and poverty. In this country it has been spread because of the promiscuity of much of the male homosexual community, the use of intravenous drugs, and increasingly the relaxed sexual morality of many contemporary heterosexuals.

This behavior is somebody's fault. All of it involves violations of inherited religious ethics, and it is engaged in by rational people, most of whom have at least a minimal awareness of the dangers they court.

The homosexual community was rife with venereal dis-

Dr. Klein

220

ease long before AIDS appeared. The hazards of drug abuse are obvious. The disasters wrought by the relaxation of sexual ethics among heterosexuals are almost too numerous to mention: teen-age pregnancy, abortion, the highest divorce rate in the Western world, the increasing impoverishment of single mothers and children, etc.

I am not so foolish as to suggest that some return to traditional morals will solve all these probelms [sic]. It is, however, equally irresponsible and foolish to imagine that there is a technological fix available for these problems as long as we don't get ourselves tangled up in the language of morality and religion.

AIDS has reminded us once again and most cruelly that sex is a matter of high seriousness. It is not a consumer good. It is — and here goes another of modern society's favorite myths — never simply a personal matter.

Sex is an integral part of marriage, family, community, and even the public health. Pretending that it is not also an area of morality and responsibility can be literally suicidal.

People are dying because of these myths. The HLTV virus has a lot of help. There is blame enough to go around, and some must surely be assigned to those who spread the dangerous, life-threatening myth that no one is to blame.

Dr. Leonard Klein, York, Pennsylvania

Sexual Perversion

So far, men who persist in the promiscuous use of the lower digestive tract as a sexual organ have been paying a price in AIDS or the fear of AIDS, and the number of AIDS victims has been doubling annually in the United States.

Jeffrey Hart, Syndicated Column (January 11, 1986).

Homos Unfaithful to Lovers

The sodomite tries to give the impression that homosexuals are not promiscuous, that they meet, fall in love like normal people, buy a house in the suburbs, park matching Volvos in the driveway, and settle down for a lifetime. Now *that* is a fairy story. Homosexuals never have a lasting relationship. Even those few who do live together for a few years are "unfaithful" to their "lovers." Their longest "marriages" last an average two or three years. But they don't *want* a lasting relationship, according to the Kinsey report. About 60 percent of the sodomites told Kinsey that they would not want a monogamous relationship. And the facts prove that they get what they want — 1,000 partners in a lifetime, according to Kinsey! The *Village Voice* has reported that 1,600 partners is more likely the more accurate number!

With such outrageous promiscuity, no wonder the AIDS curse is spreading geometrically. If you double a penny each day, you will have over $2 million in 30 days, and AIDS is exploding the same way.

Kinsey Report

900 Contacts

A 40-year-old homosexual man was initially assessed for generalized lymphadenopathy of eight months' duration. He had been in good health until July 1982 ... His medical history included an anal fistula repair, syphilis three times,

JAMA (June 21, 1985).

gonorrhea ten times, and hepatitis B. He had frequently used cocaine, amphetamines, LSD, marijuana, and amyl nitrite. He described approximately 900 anonymous sexual contacts in the past ...

R. Burkes, M.D./A. Gal, M.D./M. Stewart, M.D./P. Gill, M.D./W. Abo, M.D./M. Levin, M.D., *JAMA — (Journal of American Medical Association)*: "Simultaneous Occurrence [sic] of Pneumocystis Carinii Pneumonia, Cytomegalovirus Infection, Kaposi' Sarcoma, and B-Immunoblastic Sarcoma in a Homosexual Man" (June 21, 1985), Vol. 253 No. 23.

10,000 Contacts in a Lifetime

According to Dr. Kinsey, the average homosexual has 1,000 sex partners in a lifetime. *Village Voice* put the figure at 1,600. One activist has said that 10,000 sex partners in the lifetime of a "very active" homosexual would not be extraordinary.

Patrick J. Buchanan/J. Gordon Muir, *The American Spectator*: "Gay Times and Diseases" (August 1984), Vol. 17 No. 8, p. 1.

Sick! Sick! Sick!

The gays who got AIDS, it turned out, had often had many more sex (a lifetime average of 1,100) partners than the controls (500 partners). Not surprisingly, they had common venereal diseases like syphilis, gonorrhea and herpes, as well as the cluster of viral, bacterial and parasitic disorders that make up what is known as the "gay bowel syndrome." In addition, many AIDS patients had used amyle nitrites, the sexually stimulating inhalants called "poppers" that have been shown to produce immunosuppression.

J. Seligmann/M. Gosnell/V. Coppola/M. Hager, *Newsweek*: "The AIDS Epidemic — The Search for a Cure" (April 18, 1983).

Sexual Perversion

"Being Gay Means Doing What I Want Sexually"

Groups at highest risk for acquiring AIDS continue to be homosexual or bisexual men ... The data generated in this study were motivated by two concerns: to determine whether gay men's sexual behavior had changed since the onset of AIDS ... and to understand the factors influencing sexual behavior ...

A full 92-96% asserted they were still not taking the most basic prophylactic measures to reduce transmission and exposure to AIDS infection ...

81% of the men who agreed with the statement; "I use hot anonymous sex to relieve tension" had three or more partners the prior month ...

35% of those who agreed that reducing their number of partners would reduce their risk of AIDS had sex with more than five partners the month prior to the sampling ...

69% of the men having three or more sexual partners the previous month agreed with the statement, "It is hard to change my sexual behavior because being gay means doing what I want sexually."

L. McKusick, M.S./W. Horstman, Ph.D./T. Coates, Ph.D., *American Journal of Public Health*: "AIDS and Sexual Behavior Reported by Gay Men in San Francisco" (May 1985), Vol. 75 No. 5.

Multiple Ejaculations Daily

In the past ten years, homosexuals have asserted a right to self-expression and there has been an outburst of pent-up feeling and an overactive sexuality. Many homosexuals have more than 60 partners per year, a great preoccupation with sex, and an overactive use of masturbation, often with multiple ejaculations each day.

Robert G. Weiner, M.D., MPH, *JAMA — (Journal of the American Medical Association)*: "AIDS and Zinc Deficiency" (1984), Vol. 252.

Bathhouses and Orgies

Said Michael Callen, co-founder of Gay Men with AIDS:
"I know a gay (with AIDS) who would check into
the bathhouses Friday night & not check out until
Monday morning. In his conversations with us, he
probably had 5,000 sex partners in his life. He told
government researchers he'd only had two. He said to
us, 'You think I'm going to tell them I was a slut? I'll
go to my grave first.' "

Barton Gallman, *The Washington Post*: "Tracing AIDS Cases Raises
Privacy Issue" (July 18, 1983).

Bathhouses and Orgies
Kinky Sex

But ads for kinky and unrestrained sex still abound in the
subculture's journals. Some remaining bathhouse owners
... continue to promote such potential AIDS middens as
"orgy rooms."

D. Gelman/P. Abramson/G. Raine/P. McAlevy/P. McKillop,
Newsweek: "The Social Fallout From an Epidemic" (August 12, 1985).

Dens of Iniquity

Dr. James Oleske is a pediatrician .... "We were the first
to see AIDS in children, because our population (in
Newark) was heavy into drug abuse. One of the biggest cul-
prits in the spread of the virus may be bisexual men who go
over to the New York City bathhouses, but live in Newark
with a wife and children. Bathhouses are dens of inequity
[sic] — they're places where infections spread."

Giovanna Breu, *People*: "Aids: Fatal, Incurable and Spreading" (June
17, 1985).

Sexual Perversion

"I Want Fun While I Tick"

The only place where there seems to be conversation is at the lunch counter, where two naked men are munching on hamburgers and talking about the AIDS (acquired immune deficiency syndrome) epidemic that has terrified the city. "I could get back into the closet right now," says one of the men, "and still get it in a year or so. So what would I have achieved? Celibacy." The other nods enthusiastically "I know," he says. "We're just little time bombs, aren't we?" Then he stands, stretches, and wipes his mouth with a napkin. "Well, I don't know about you, but I'm going to have some fun while I tick."

Peter Collier/David Horowitz, *California Magazine*: "Whitewash" (July 1983).

Midnight in the Gay World

"For a moment, I remember the first night I waked with night sweats and listened to the raucous sounds of the French Quarter, where men were still out before dawn, willfully threatening themselves with exposure to an incurable disease.

"... I know men are still out on the streets of the French Quarter — the streets of America — testing their fates against the virus ... The never-ending midnight of the gay world will continue until AIDS has claimed the last dancer in the last disco. I have danced in those discos from London to New York to San Francisco ..."

Johnny Greene, *People*: "A Writer Fights a Faceless Enemy and Learns To Live With Fear" (June 17, 1985).

Legalizing Perversion for 14 Year Olds: The Election on September 10th Is Crucial for the Future of the Province of Ontario

The citizens of Ontario have an excellent opportunity to send a clear message to Mr. Peterson, the Premier of Ontario and Mr. Rae, the leader of the New Democratic Party, who by signing the NDP-Liberal Accord in 1985 created the governing majority.

The most infamous accomplishment of the Peterson government certainly was the "Sexual Orientation" amendment to the Ontario Human Rights Code of Bill 7 which gave homosexuals, lesbians and people of other sexual perversion legal status and special rights.

Thus we have the affliction of sexual orientation in Ontario, which is a vague undefined and open-ended idea. Not only would it extend legal support to homosexual behavior, but could open the door to other types of behavior, which could then in turn be legalized by changes to the Federal Criminal Code. It should be noted in this context that Svend Robinson, a federal NDP member has offered an amendment to the criminal code to lower the age of consent for anal intercourse to fourteen years.

Ontario Political Action Committee

(Could this kind of perversion be the reason I was so viciously attacked by pro gay media people in this city? — JVI)

Sexual Promiscuity

Sexual Promiscuity Destroys Civilizations

John D. Unwin, a British anthropologist who has spent years studying the rise and fall of 80 civilizations has concluded that no society can long endure widespread sexual promiscuity.

He found that all of the cultures he studied followed a similar sexual pattern. During its early days of existence, premarital and extramarital sexual relationships were strictly prohibited. This period coincided with great creative energy, causing the culture to prosper.

Much later, people began to rebel against the prohibitions, demanding freedom. As the morals weakened, social energy abated — eventually resulting in the decay or destruction of the civilization.

"Any human society is free to choose either to display great energy, or to enjoy sexual freedom; the evidence is that they cannot do both for more than one generation."

"The Flaming Torch"

Why U.S. Leads in Teen Pregnancy

The shocking prevalence of teenage pregnancy among white as well as black Americans was brought to light earlier this year, when the Alan Guttmacher Institute, a nonprofit research center in New York City, released the results of a 37-country study. Its findings: the U.S. leads nearly all other developed nations in its incidence of pregnancy involving teens ages 15 through 19 ....

To understand the nature of the problem, one must look beyond statistics and examine the dramatic changes in attitudes and social mores that have swept through American culture over the past 30 years ....

Social workers are almost unanimous in citing the influ-

Time Magazine (December 9, 1985).

ence of the popular media — television, rock music, videos, movies — in propelling the trend toward precocious sexuality. One survey has shown that in the course of a year the average viewer sees more than 9,000 scenes of suggested sexual intercourse or innuendo on prime-time TV. "Our young people are barraged by the message that to be sophisticated they must be sexually hip," says Williams. "They don't even buy toothpaste to clean their teeth. They buy it to be sexually attractive."

Time Magazine (December 9, 1985).

Sexually Transmitted Diseases

The World Health Organization (WHO) has estimated there are between 30 million and 50 million cases of venereal syphilis in the world and more than 150 million cases of gonorrhea infection. Director general of the WHO, Halfdon Mahler, estimates there may be 10 million carriers of the AIDS virus in the world's population.

During the 1960s gonococcus organisms became increasingly drug resistant. Then during the 1970s genital herpes swiftly cut through the ranks of the sexually permissive.

In the West in the 1980s, AIDS, caused by the HTLV-3 virus, swept first through homosexual ranks. It was then spread by bisexuals to heterosexuals, who in turn spread it to their mates or partners.

Donald D. Schroeder, World Health Organization News Release

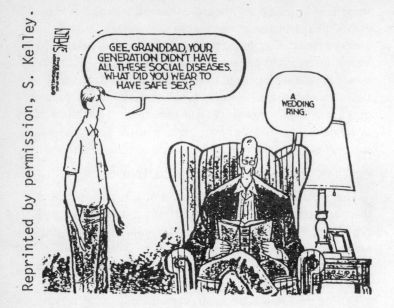

3,000 Years of Sex Scourges

It was Moses who started the war on STD's, back when his soldiers came home from defeating the Midianites and brought with them thousands of captive women. He quickly saw a problem — "a plague among the congregation" — and acted. He invoked a one-week quarantine and condemned "every woman that hath known man by lying with him."

Some 3,000 years and many sex plagues later — in fact up till the 1900s — even skilled physicians didn't know what to do about STD's. Many didn't want to know. To treat a sex disease, they felt, was to sanction sin.

STD's maimed kings, queens and Popes plus chunks of

U.S. News & World Report (June 2, 1986).

armies, navies and cities. Victims in the past 100 years ranged from Adolf Hitler and Al Capone to Oscar Wilde and Wild Bill Hickok.

More than once, history was altered. Sixteenth-century Russia had been put on a progressive path by an enlightened Ivan IV until syphilis turned him into Ivan the Terrible.

STD origins have long been debated. After syphilis swept Europe in the 1490s, many called it the Naples disease. The English termed it French pox. Some French knew it as the Spanish disease, claiming that Columbus's crew carried it from America to Spain — an issue still in dispute.

Cure after cure was tried. German men in the 15th century hoped to purge syphilis in bathhouses, but nude women did the scrubbing and the disease multiplied. The year 1900 found Americans relying on Unfortunate's Friend and other quack remedies laced with alcohol.

To keep men fit for World War I, the U.S. detained up to 30,000 prostitutes in camps, many with barbed wire, reports Harvard historian Allan Brandt — a move akin to the interning of Japanese Americans in World War II.

Major progress came in 1938 when Congress funded local venereal-disease-control programs. Soon, every state was requiring blood tests for marriage licenses.

Only 5 percent of draftees entered World War II with VD, compared with 13 percent reporting for World War I. "Knock out VD" was a '40s slogan, and penicillin's debut in 1944 nearly did.

But STD's never die. Diseases change and require new cures, notes Brandt. "It's a constant problem keeping up with the microbes that are on this planet."

Sexual Promiscuity

What Are Your Chances of Getting AIDS From Sexual Contact?

Eight Years Abstinence To Be Sure

If you a heterosexual male, you can get AIDS from an infected female partner. Vaginal secretions may contain the AIDS virus, which can infect you through small openings in the skin.

If you are a heterosexual female, the virus in an infected partner's semen can enter your bloodstream through even the smallest tear in the vaginal wall — or rectum wall, if you engage in anal sex.

If you are a homosexual male, the virus can enter your bloodstream during anal sex with an infected partner. The rectum wall is very susceptible to tearing during sex, so you could be infected by both blood and semen.

If you are a homosexual female, you can get AIDS through contact with an infected female partner's vaginal secretions.

Because the virus exists in its most potent form in semen and in blood, sexual contact is one of the two major ways to contact AIDS.

This means that people with multiple male and female sex partners, men who have sex with prostitutes and men who have sexual contact with other men are at high risk for AIDS. (High risk individuals should always use a condom when having sex. A spermicide containing nonoxynol-9 may add extra protection — researchers believe it may help destroy the AIDS virus.)

Conversely, if you have no sexual contact or are in a completely monogamous relationship, you are at no or very low risk for AIDS. But because symptoms of AIDS can take years after infection to appear, abstinence or fidelity is no protection unless it has lasted eight years.

Detroit News (January 10, 1988).

One Affair Could Involve Hundreds

Health and Human Services Secretary Otis R. Bowen: "So remember when a person has sex, they're not just having sex with that partner, they're having it with everybody that partner had it with for the past 10 years."

Billings Gazette: "Millions May Die From AIDS" (Associated Press, January 3, 1987) p. 1.

American Red Cross Warns the Public

You are at risk for getting AIDS and spreading the AIDS virus if —

- You are a man who has had sex with another man since 1977, **even one time**.
- You have ever taken illegal drugs by needle.
- You are a native of Haiti, Burundi, Kenya, Rwanda, Tanzania, Uganda, or Zaire who entered the United States after 1977.
- You have AIDS or one of its signs or symptoms.
- You have ever had a positive test for HTLV-III antibody, showing past exposure to the AIDS virus.
- You have hemophilia and have received clotting factor concentrates.
- You are or have been the sex partner of any person described above since 1977.
- You are a woman or man who is now or has been a prostitute since 1977.
- You have been the heterosexual sex partner of a male or female prostitute within the last six months.

American Red Cross

Sexual Transmission

Koop Speaks

How Exposed

Although the AIDS virus is found in several body fluids, a person acquires the virus during sexual contact with an infected person's blood or semen and possibly vaginal secretions. The virus then enters a person's blood stream through their rectum, vagina or penis.

Small (unseen by the naked eye) tears in the surface lining of the vagina or rectum may occur during insertion of the penis, fingers, or other objects, thus opening an avenue for entrance of the virus directly into the blood stream; therefore, the AIDS virus can be passed from penis to rectum and vagina and vice versa without a visible tear in the tissue or the presence of blood.

Prevention of Sexual Transmission — Know Your Partner

Couples who maintain mutually faithful monogamous relationships (only one continuing sexual partner) are protected from AIDS through sexual transmission. If you have been faithful for at least five years and your partner has been faithful too, neither of you is at risk. If you have not been faithful, then you and your partner are at risk. If your partner has not been faithful, then your partner is at risk which also puts you at risk. This is true for both heterosexual and homosexual couples. Unless it is possible to know with *absolute certainty* that neither you nor your sexual partner is carrying the virus of AIDS, you must use protective behavior. *Absolute certainty* means not only that you and your partner have maintained a mutually faithful monogamous sexual relationship, but it means that neither you nor your partner has used illegal intravenous drugs.

Surgeon General Koop's pamphlet on AIDS

Is the Medical Profession Really Protecting the Public From AIDS?

Dr. Stephen Joseph, New York City's health commissioner, has broken ranks with many of his spineless colleagues in the medical profession and is calling on his state legislature to enact laws that would require doctors to inform the sex partners of patients who carry the AIDS virus.

He is concerned about the 1,005 women who his city health department says have contracted AIDS — many of whom did not know that their spouses or sex partners were infected. Many couples both use the same doctor. Is not the physician of the woman just as responsible in such cases as the spouse, if he knows her spouse is infected, to warn her in advance that relations with her husband may destroy her life?

Will it take a lawsuit against her doctor to force the medical profession to protect themselves by warning patients who live with AIDS carriers of the risk they are taking?

The ACLU has announced that "it sees no conflict between civil liberties and sound public health policies." In other words, they see no reason why doctors should inform their patients' partners about their sexual hazard. They ought to try telling that to the 1,005 women who will soon die because they were not warned to protect themselves.

Isn't it time the medical profession and government leaders pay more attention to protecting the healthy members of society than those who defy the laws of God and man?

Dr. Tim LaHaye, *Capital Report* (Fall 1987).

Terrorism

Blood and Sexual Terrorism

Robert Schwab, a homosexual activist dying of AIDS and late President of the Texas Human Rights Foundation, stated: "There has come the idea that if research money (for AIDS) is not forth coming at a certain level by a certain date, that all gay males should give blood ... whatever action is required to get national attention is valid. If that includes blood terrorism, so be it."

Dallas Gay News, "Special Report: AIDS" (Noebel/Cameron/Lutton, May 20, 1983).

"I Will Take Others to the Grave With Me"

Some people infected with the AIDS virus are so filled with "rage" and the desire to "get back at the world" that they continue sexual activity, knowing that they might give the deadly disease to others, local and national experts say.

"I've talked to some people with such tremendous rage at being infected with HIV (the AIDS virus) that they've vowed to get even," Martha Gross, a Washington sex therapist said in an interview.

"They say things like, 'I'm only 29 and I'm going to die. It's just not fair.' They make up their minds they will take other victims with them," she said.

Joyce Price, *The Washington Times* (November 6, 1987).

"I've got gay cancer. I'm going to die, and so are you."

— Ex post facto announcement reportedly made to sexual conquests by the late Gaetan Dugas, a homosexual French Canadian airline steward who may have been the person to first bring the AIDS virus to the United States, when he came to New York in 1976 for the visit of the Tall Ships — whose story is told in a new book, entitled *And the Band Played On: Politics, People and the AIDS Epidemic.*

"I Want to Take Others With Me"

Dr. John Dwyer, the former Chief of Immunology at Yale-New Haven Hospital who has treated more than 400 patients, says: "Every now and then, there are people who say, 'I know I'm going to die and I'm going to take as many people with me as I can.' "

Dr. John Dwyer, Chief of Immunology, Yale-New Haven Hospital.

Stop Typhoid Marys

"Gays put pressure on the Board of Health to forbid the test," says Kaplan [Dr. Helen Singer Kaplan] of the Human Sexuality Program at the New York Hospital-Cornell Medical Center. "We could stop the spread of AIDS today if these high-risk people, these Typhoid Marys, would stop spreading the disease. As a physician and a scientist, I'm appalled at their wildly having sex and spreading AIDS."

J. H. Tanne, *New York Magazine*: "The Last Word on Avoiding AIDS" (October 7, 1985).

AIDS Victim Arrested

Sexual Terrorist

A 45-year-old former United States Army sergeant, suspected of knowingly spreading AIDS to his sexual partners, has been arrested in Nuremberg, West Germany.

The *New York Times* reported on February 21, that the American, whose name has been withheld, will be charged under a law that prohibits causing "bodily harm" with a weapon or "dangerous treatment."

Under the West German penal code, the man could be sentenced to five years in prison.

A spokesman at the American Consulate in Munich said American officials have contacted the retired sergeant, who is the first person ever arrested in the Bavarian state for spreading the sexual disease.

Doug Waymire, *New York Times*

Terrorism

"AIDS Is My Strength"

"Don't call us AIDS victims. AIDS is not my weakness. AIDS is my strength."

Ralph Diamond, a homosexual activist with AIDS

"We Will Sodomize Your Sons"

Homosexual activist Michael Swift writing in Boston's Gay Community News of February 15, 1987 asserts in his essay, "For the Homoerotic Order": "We [homosexuals] shall sodomize your sons ... we shall seduce them in your schools, in your dormitories, in your gymnasiums, in your locker rooms, in your sports arenas, in your seminaries, in your youth groups, in your movie theater bathrooms, in your army bunkhouses, in your truck stops, in your all male clubs, in your houses of congress ... your sons will do our bidding. They will be recast in our image. They will come to crave and adore us."

Michael Swift, *Gay Community News* (February 15, 1987).

Mass Murderers

Sodomites are the most vicious people in the world. Many of the mass murders have been committed by sodomites. They don't like to talk of mass homosexual killers like Dean Coril, Elmer Henley, Jr., John Gacy, William Bonin, Bruce Davis, Wayne Williams, Henry Lucas, Otis Toole, etc. Out of 518 deaths in the past 17 years, sodomites killed 350 of them — 68 percent (and remember that homosexuals make up only about 4 percent of the population).

Some of the most extensive torture-mass-murders of the twentieth century were performed by three homosexual rapists — a Texas engineer, the California Trash Bag murderer, and the Chicago contractor. In these cases, aggression was repeated and premeditated, and it included torture, homo-

Dr. Dumas, *Gay Is Not Good.*

sexual rape, mutilation or dismemberment, and murder. In each case there were about thirty murders of boys and young men.

Dr. Dumas, *Gay Is Not Good*

Children Stolen to Satisfy Cravings

Due to the tremendous increase in the overt homosexual population and because the young male child is a favored sexual object of many homosexuals, thousands of children are stolen from parents to meet the sexual needs of homosexuals. The seductions to which these abducted children are subjected stunt their sexual growth and, not unusually, they develop into perverts. Consequently, few ever seek their way home again.

Dr. Melvin Anchell, M.D., *The New American*: "A Doctor Looks at Homosexuality" (March 17, 1986).

Testing and Legislation for AIDS

Legislation

Health is ... the focus of AIDS legislation introduced in the 100th Congress by Representative William Dannemeyer (R-CA).

House resolution 338 would "make it a federal offense for certain persons to intentionally donate blood, semen or an organ" if the person knew he:

(1) has acquired immune deficiency syndrome,

(2) has had sexual relations with a male since January 1, 1977,

(3) is an intravenous drug user,

(4) received a blood transfusion within the past year, is a hemophiliac who has used a clotting factor, or

(5) has engaged in prostitution since January 1, 1977.

The legislation requires that: "any person who violates this Act shall be subject to imprisonment for not more than 10 years."

If passed, another piece of AIDS legislation would express the wish of Congress that each state enact certain laws pertaining to AIDS.

House Concurrent Resolution 8 would encourage each of the 50 states to pass laws including:

- Legislation that would require all person who are seeking a marriage license to be tested for AIDS or the virus known as HTLV-III/LAV.

- Legislation that would require the tracing of individuals with venereal disease to include individuals with AIDS, AIDS Complex, or the virus which causes AIDS.

- Legislation that would encourage designated hospitals to offer blood transfusions which are made directly between the blood donor and person receiving the

Education Reporter (February 1987).

transfusion.

- Legislation that would permit nurses to wear protective garments at their discretion when dealing with individuals who have AIDS.

Education Reporter: "Legislation Update: What's on the 1987 Agenda" (February 1987), No. 13.

Official Recommendations

NOTE: The following 15 specific recommendations are put forward by the National AIDS Prevention Institute as measures intended to help counteract the lethal AIDS epidemic. It is hoped that these recommendations will stimulate discussion and debate, and encourage constructive action for the protection of human life.

1. *Separation of Public Health Policy and Politics.* Due recognition of the unique value of human life demands the consistent application of proven scientific methods for combatting any and all epidemics of infectious diseases. Scientifically established life-protective measures must be implemented for effective counteraction of all disease, at all times, in all parts of the country, wholly uninfluenced and unmodified by political considerations which may be raised by various special interest groups from time to time. AIDS must be depoliticized.

2. *Blood screening determined by scientific considerations.* In the interest of protecting as many human lives as possible, the voluntary or mandatory blood testing of some or all U.S. citizens and foreign persons entering or residing in the U.S.A. should be undertaken as widely and as frequently as required by scientific/epidemiological considerations, wholly apart from political factors.

3. *Pre-marital blood screening.* Blood testing for antibodies to the AIDs retrovirus (HIV) as a pre-requisite for issuance of marriage licenses nation-wide.

4. *Confidential contact tracing.* Complete confidential contact tracing wherever test results are positive — to

National AIDS Prevention Institute

include free testing of all former sex partners and blood recipients of the infected person.

5. *Appropriate follow-up on antibody positive persons.* All persons determined through whatever screening programs, to be antibody positive for the AIDS retrovirus, must be reported confidentially to public health departments and given the benefit of the best medical care available plus thorough education as to how best to avoid transmission of their infection to others.

6. *Restraint of infected persons as a last resort where necessary.* In order to curb the spread of the AIDS epidemic and to save as many lives as possible, those antibody positive persons who fail to respond appropriately to educational and counseling programs must be segregated or restrained by whatever means are necessary to assure non-transmission of infection to others.

7. *Autologous and directed blood donations.* Autologous and directed donations of blood at the option of the donor and donee, to include the requirement that all such blood be subjected to full screening for antibodies to the AIDS retrovirus and for detection of other health-threatening infectious agents.

8. *Educational courses on AIDS.* A course of study on AIDS in every High School, College and University in the nation, presenting the facts concerning the AIDS retrovirus, its transmission, and prevention of infection through the safest of all methods — limitation of sexual activity to marriage.

9. *A truth campaign concerning the unreliability of condoms.* A study conducted by scientists at the University of Miami Medical Center found that three

National AIDS Prevention Institute

out of ten infected persons transmitted AIDS infection to their sex partner in spite of the use of condoms exclusively in all sexual activities. Rational individuals who value their life will readily conclude that a 30% risk of infection by a lethal retrovirus is unacceptable. All public health officials agree that the use of condoms will not eliminate the risk of infection. The American public must be told the truth about the demonstrated unreliability of condoms as barriers to transmission of HIV.

10. *Limitation of sexual activity to marriage.* The safest of all sexual activity is that which takes place exclusively between uninfected persons within the framework of responsibility defined by monogamous marriage.

11. *Screening of individuals convicted of engaging in prostitution.* All persons arrested and convicted on charges of female or male prostitution should be tested for the presence of antibodies to the retrovirus which causes AIDS. Whatever measures are necessary must be taken to assure that such persons do not continue to work as prostitutes.

12. *Closure of public centers of on-site sexual activities.* All bath houses and other public facilities in which on-site sexual activities occur must be closed at once.

13. *Screening of health care workers and food handlers.* All physicians, nurses, dentists, other personal-contact health care workers and food handlers should be screened for antibodies to the AIDS retrovirus at such intervals as scientific considerations would prescribe, and those testing positive should be barred from continuation of such services.

14. *Screening of persons entering detention facilities.* All persons entering detention facilities, jails and prisons

National AIDS Prevention Institute

of all kinds should be subjected to blood screening, and those who are confirmed positive to AIDS virus antibodies should be segregated throughout their incarceration period, given appropriate health care, educated and followed up subsequent to their release.

15. *Right of employers to terminate services of infected persons*. Employers who are concerned that the attack of HIV on the brain of infected employees may render such employees incompetent and/or hazardous to the lives of others, should be free to terminate the employment of persons known to be infected by HIV.

National AIDS Prevention Institute, Scientific Advisors: Gordon M. Dickinson, M.D., *Infectious Diseases*, W. Daniel Jordan, M.D., *Vascular Surgeon*, Paul E. Kaldahl, M.D., *Pathologist*, Mark I. Klein, M.D., *Psychiatrist*, Vernon H. Mark, M.D., *Neurologist*, Alton Ochsner, M.D., *Cardiologist and Surgeon*, Lawrence B. Sandberg, M.D., Ph.D., *Pathologist*, Gwendolyn B. Scott, M.D., *Pediatric Infectious Diseases*, Frank G. Simon, M.D., *Allergy and Internal Medicine*, James I. Slaff, M.D., *Gastroenterologist*.

The Right To Know About AIDS

We live in a time of madness, a time when public and private foolishness reigns. We have among us a plague, a disease so deadly that anyone who is contaminated will most likely die. The official estimate is that one to two million Americans are carriers of this plague; some estimates run as high as four million. We can observe two hundred Americans and know that, mathematically, one is a deadly transmitter of the AIDS virus and poses a threat to us all.

But the "one" who is contaminated is unidentified. Why? Because the law protects AIDS carriers from disclosing their identity, thereby concealing the magnitude of the problem. Imagine that, a deadly disease with civil rights.

In California, the madness is complete. A doctor is restricted by law from informing another doctor that a referred patient has AIDS. Legally, doctors cannot tell hospital nurses, or any health care provider who may come in contact with the infected person, that his patient has AIDS. A doctor can't even inform the spouse of an infected individual. What monumental ignorance, what dangerous superciliousness, what deadly logic; murder in the name of privacy!

How would you, the reader, like to work in a hospital emergency clinic and participate in the care of incoming patients, often bloody and dirty, without knowing if the AIDS virus is present? How about the patient? How does he know that the doctor hasn't been infected at some prior time? What about the dental hygienist? It is not work without its share of blood. Plaque may not be the only enemy to both patient and hygienist. Do we not have a right to know if someone is a carrier of AIDS?

Doctors of all categories have hundreds of patients; their

Richardson, *The Forerunner* (September 1987).

exposure to AIDS is guaranteed. When my grandchildren visit the dentist or physician, I am reasonably assured that they have treated an AIDS patient unknowingly. Could they be infected? Chances of accidental infection are greater than the average. How about an obstetrician or a gynecologist?

Americans shouldn't kid themselves. Doctors are discussing the possibilities of their personal infection. It is becoming a factor in early retirement for members of the medical community, and, as the problem gets worse, we will have fewer doctors to treat the disease.

American lawmakers should be debating how we should test all adult Americans, not, if we should test. Since studies show that 85 percent of those who carry the HIV virus (Human Immunodeficiency Virus) also called the AIDS virus are unaware they have it, our public policy must promote widespread testing. Carriers must be made aware of the fact they have the disease so they will avoid infecting others. Actually, they could be murdering others without even knowing it; studies have shown people can be carriers for 10-15 years without any symptoms.

Our medical authorities desperately need to know who is and who is not a carrier. We need to get on with the testing as soon as possible. Every day that passes without testing exacerbates the problem. It's time for the State Department of Health to devise a plan for mandatory state testing. It's going to happen, but it's only a matter of time, courage and leadership.

Senator H. L. Richardson, *The Forerunner*: "Richardson Report" (September 1987) p. 11.

Testing for AIDS

Testing

It is unquestionably clear that we have to take immediate measures for wide spread public health testing.

Dr. Vernon A. Mark, Associate Professor of Surgery, Harvard Medical School, Interview with Dr. Ed Rowe, President, New National AIDS Prevention Institute (March 1987).

Mandatory Testing

Secretary of Education William J. Bennett says all people should undergo mandatory AIDS blood tests before they are admitted to a hospital, enter or leave prison, marry or seek to immigrate to the United States.

News Record: "Widespread AIDS Tests Supported by Bennett" (Associated Press, May 3, 1987).

Stupidity Is In

Just six months ago it was only folks with a right-wing agenda who were talking about routine testing for AIDS. Now the *New England Journal of Health* is recognizing that it's stupid to be trying to combat the disease without knowing the extent of it.

Gary Bauer, Domestic Policy Advisor to the President/T. Morganthau/ M. G. Warner/M. Hager, *Newsweek*: "Facing the AIDS Crisis" (June 8, 1987).

One Has a Right to Know

The AMA's Schwartz says: "When someone has the potential of transmitting the disease to someone who isn't infected, the second party has the right to know. When that happens, society cancels out individual rights and opts for what is good for the society at large."

J. Carey/B. Quick/R. Riley, *U.S. News & World Report*: "A Time of Testing: AIDS" (April 20, 1987), p. 58.

Playing With Death

Sen. Bill Armstrong [R., Colorado] introduced legislation to overturn a Supreme Court ruling that extended anti-discrimination protection for handicapped people to include victims of contagious diseases such as AIDS.

"The court's ruling raises legal obstacles to removing someone with a contagious disease," said Armstrong.

"This will put parents, school children, employers and employees in a terrible situation.

"It's simply irresponsible to permit people with a deadly disease to infect others," Armstrong said.

(Associated Press, March 7, 1987).

Tolerance for Perversion

Today's humanitarian effort to understand and sympathize with those unfortunate individuals who have become perverted is commendable, but it has gone overboard in a tolerance for perversion that has left the normal individual unprotected. As a result, children and adults are becoming contaminated to an alarming degree ....

It is time for humanitarian concern to swing away from the pervert and direct sympathy and efforts towards rescuing the victims.

Dr. Melvin Anchell, M.D. and Psychiatrist

No Rights When Dead

Dr. Phillip Reiff of San Francisco's Castro Medical Clinic: "I get tired of some in the gay community complaining about how testing invades their civil rights, because you don't have any [rights] when you're dead."

T. Monmaney/P. Wingert/G. Raine/M. Gosnell, *Newsweek*: "AIDS: Who Should Be Tested" (May 11, 1987).

Right To Live

National Hemophilia Foundation advisor Louis Aledort, M.D., of Mount Sinai Medical Center in New York, ... told *JAMA* Medical News: "I disagree vehemently with the National Gay Task Force. They may want, to protect their rights, but what about the hemophiliacs' right to life?"

William A. Check, Ph.D., *JAMA — (Journal of American Medical Association)*: "Preventing AIDS Transmission: Should Blood Donors Be Screened?" (1983), Vol. 249.

Theories

*I have literally read hundreds upon hundreds of articles on AIDS. Some of these dealt with theories on the origin of this virus. I studied **Who Murdered Africa**, by William Campbell Douglas, M.D., **The Great AIDS Hoax**, by T. C. Fry, that deals with the poisoning and destruction of the body by AIDS via the eating of junk foods. I also read Stoner's racist presentation that places the blame for AIDS on Jews and blacks, plus C. B. Baker's report on AIDS being a communist conspiracy as the Soviets beam electromagnetic warfare against the United States. Such action he claims generates gene mutations and causes dormant viruses to suddenly become attack killers.*

May I caution one and all to be very suspicious on such reports. Instead, stay with the facts as presented in this book by myriads of trained specialists. Don't become sidetracked by one eccentric. In a multitude of counselors there is safety. Thus I have avoided the wildfire reports of a few and presented the statements of multiplied experts as has undoubtedly been discovered by readers at this point. — JVI

Vaccines

No Cure — No Hope

A cure for AIDS, or even a vaccine to prevent its further spread, now seem like distant goals, despite earlier optimism, officials say. "As an optimist, I will tell you I am not expecting a cure," Koop said.

Paul Raeburn, *News Record*: "Fear of AIDS Strikes Rural Areas" (Associated Press, May 6, 1987).

One Hundred Percent Fatal

The reason we call AIDS a "dreaded disease" is that it is 100 percent fatal, and it is possible that a vaccine will never be found to cure it.

Dr. James McKeever, Ph.D., *The AIDS Plague*, p. 45.

Multiple Strains

Dr. David Cohn of Denver Disease Control says that it's basically unrealistic to talk about a cure for AIDS "because of the unusual way the AIDS virus multiplies within the lymph cells, every case can potentially be a different strain." So the problem of multiple strains makes a cure and a vaccine almost impossible.

Dr. David Cohn, Denver Disease Control

Rapid Reproduction

As the (AIDS) virus replicates (reproduces itself) it evolves rapidly so that there are always many immunologically different strains present in an infected individual. This is one of the reasons that it has not been possible to produce vaccines and that it may not be possible to do so even in theory. While we may hope for a miraculous cure, it is not likely.

A.D.J. Robertson, President, Research Testing & Development Corp., Lexington, Georgia.

Swift Spreading Disease

Dr. Hazeltine [sic] of Harvard says: "Trying to develop a vaccine for AIDS is like trying to hit a moving target.

Dr. J. Slaff/J. Brubaker, *The AIDS Epidemic*, p. 186.

Destruction of Brain Cells

The AIDS virus belongs to the family of lentiviruses; it is not, as was thought first, a human leukemia virus. These retroviruses cause several diseases in domestic animals, including infectious anemia in horses and encephalitis in goats. They cannot be treated and it has proven impossible to develop vaccines; infected animals must be slaughtered. AIDS is a set of symptoms which have been narrowly defined by the Centers for Disease Control. The AIDS virus causes further symptoms not included in the CDC definition because, like the other known lentiviruses, it infects primarily the central nervous system, becoming incorporated in the genetic material of brain cells, but also being expressed as replicating virions in blood and brain tissue. As the virus replicates it evolves rapidly so that there are always many immunologically different strains present in an infected individual. This is one of the reasons that it has not been possible to produce vaccines and that it may not be possible to prevent viral replication in the blood — and there is no reason to suppose that it is — such a therapy would have to be continued for life because it could not destroy the retroviral DNA incorporated in the genome of brain cells without destroying the brain cells themselves.

A.D.J. Robertson, *The Wall Street Journal*: "The Virulence of AIDS" (October 31, 1985).

Vaccines

Vaccines May Have Triggered the World's Greatest Plague

AIDS: Another Look

Dr. Robert Mendelsohn, M.D., writing in his newsletter *The People's Doctor*, reports that Dr. Robert Gallo (the U.S. expert who first identified the AIDS virus) now believes there may be a link between the UN World Health Organization smallpox eradication program and the AIDS epidemic in Africa.

"I cannot say that it actually happened," Dr. Gallo explained, "but I have been saying for some years that the use of live vaccine such as that used for smallpox can activate a dormant infection such as AIDS."

Dr. Mendelsohn, noting the extent to which drug addicts have been blamed for spreading AIDS by sharing needles, reveals that "in the recent WHO smallpox vaccination campaign, needles were reused 40-60 times." And he further notes that the AIDS epidemic matches the concentration of smallpox vaccinations in Africa and South America.

The theory that the AIDS epidemic in Africa may have been triggered by the smallpox immunization program has apparently sparked an intense behind-the-scenes debate among scientists.

"You may not have heard about this debate," Dr. Mendelsohn continues, "but an urgent call for evidence to support the idea has been demanded by the World Health Organization. This theory was discussed by WHO officials last autumn. No follow-up data are available from the smallpox eradication program because no systematic studies of the complications produced by the mass immunization have been done(!)."

An unnamed WHO advisor who first disclosed the

Daily News Digest (October 21, 1987).

problem to the *London Times* asserts: "I thought it was just a coincidence until we studied the latest findings about the reactions which can be caused by vaccinia. Now I believe the smallpox vaccine theory is the explanation to the explosion of AIDS."

Dr. Mendelsohn points out that this theory "also provides an explanation of how AIDS infection is spread more evenly between males and females in Africa than in the West." And he asserts: "Further evidence of the link between AIDS and the smallpox vaccine comes from the Walter Reed Army Medical Center in Washington, D.C., where routine smallpox vaccination of a 19-year-old Army recruit was the trigger for the stimulation of dormant HIV virus into full-blown AIDS.

This discovery was made by a medical team working with Dr. Robert Redfield at Walter Reed. The recruit developed AIDS two and one-half weeks after being immunized against smallpox, and he died shortly thereafter."

Daily News Digest (October 21, 1987), p. 4. Used by permission.

Also see "Monkeys and the AIDS-Immunization Connection" under the title "Origins of AIDS."

Too Late for Tens of Thousands

Because the typical time between infection with HIV and the development of clinical AIDS is four or more years, most of the persons who will develop AIDS between now and 1991 already are infected.

Issues in Science & Technology

AIDS Virus Multiplies 100 Times Faster Than Influenza

... the genetic characteristic of the AIDS virus and the antibody, characteristic of, the AIDS virus changes. The change occurs in the code of the AIDS virus, 100 times more rapidly than it does in the influenza virus. You've got to remember that there's some even more simple viruses that have been around a long time, for which we still do not have effective vaccines ...

Dr. Vernon A. Mark, Associate Professor of Surgery, Harvard Medical School, Interview with Dr. Ed Rowe, President, New AIDS Prevention Institute (March 1987).

180 Different AIDS Viruses and 400 Strains

Throughout the entire incubation period, the human victim is decidedly "infected" and capable of infecting others if they, through whatever means, should receive components of any of the victims' sperm or other body fluids into their blood stream.

As far as we know, AIDS is the first lentiviral disease ever to have launched an attack against the human species. "Lenti" is Latin for "slow." Because HIV is slow-working, it is highly deceptive. Millions may become infected without even knowing it — and may year-after-year transmit the killer to more and more other persons. The longer the incubation period, the greater the probability of infecting

Dr. Rowe, *CMA Newsletter* (February 1987).

numerous others — especially if the "carrier" is sexually unrestricted as a large portion of the U.S. population is ...

Not only is a lentivirus a slow actor: It's also a constantly changing one. It keeps changing its protein overcoat and presenting different faces. Five different variants have been isolated from a single strain. In Frankfurt, Germany, scientists have identified 180 "different" AIDS viruses. In Atlanta, scientists at the Centers for Disease Control (CDC) have classified over 400 variant strains of HIV.

So let's understand that this particular villain presents a constantly changing target. Take aim at him — and all of a sudden he's something else. Now he's a genetic variant that your trusty scientific "gun" can't possibly hit. No wonder even the most accomplished scientists are baffled. Heroically they pursue the enemy, but the enemy changes, changes, and changes.

Dr. Ed Rowe, President, New National AIDS Prevention Institute, *CMA Newsletter* (February 1987).

Genes of AIDS Virus Mutate One Million to Ten Million Times Faster Than the Genes of Human Beings

Always-Changing AIDS Virus Tough to Diagnose, Treat

WASHINGTON — New research suggests that the AIDS virus, which once appeared to be a manageable single entity, is a complex family of rapidly mutating viruses that like a clever enemy can constantly change its weaponry, its camouflage, its defenses and even its targets in the body.

As a result of the mutations in AIDS viruses there may be thousands of slightly different forms, some possibly having specialized abilities to be transmitted, to infect different tis-

Cincinnati Enquirer (September 8, 1987).

Viruses

sues, to evade the immune system or to resist drug treatments.

According to new findings at the Los Alamos National Laboratory ... the genes of the AIDS virus are mutating between one million and 10 million times faster than the genes of human beings.

The flu virus has taken 50 years to evolve as much as the AIDS virus has in the last 10 years, the Los Alamos study shows. New flu vaccines must be developed every few years to keep up with the changes.

Some AIDS researchers suspect that some of the variations in the AIDS virus that are already known are the result of mutations in the recent past. There is even evidence that within the lifetime of any one AIDS patient, the original strain of virus that began the infection can give rise to several new strains, all of which continue to proliferate.

The Los Alamos finding "casts bewildering shadows" across the prospects for reliable diagnosis, broadly effective treatment and a vaccine that will block all forms of the virus, Gerald Myers, a molecular geneticist who measured the rate of change at the New Mexico laboratory, said recently.

Los Alamos, better known for its research on nuclear weapons, operates a computerized AIDS virus data base. It contains the specific genetic codes, or sequences, from about 30 different AIDS viruses isolated from 1976 to 1986.

Myers suggested that if large enough changes in the AIDS virus arise, some strains could be different enough that a vaccine against one fails to protect against another. This is one of the reasons that vaccine workers are becoming pessimistic about achieving their goals soon.

For the same reasons, the AIDS antibody test could fail to detect the presence of an infection. The test looks for a spe-

Cincinnati Enquirer (September 8, 1987).

cific kind of antibody and if the person's immune system has manufactured a different one — appropriate to a mutated AIDS virus — the test could fail to detect an infection.

Cincinnati Enquirer (*The Washington Post*, September 8, 1987). Used by permission.

2nd AIDS Virus Found in U.S.

A second AIDS virus discovered 2 1/2 years ago in West Africa, and which later spread to Europe, has been found in a patient in Newark, N.J., researchers said Wednesday.

Researchers at the University of Medicine and Dentistry of New Jersey said it is the first time the virus has been seen in the Western Hemisphere. However, there was no evidence that the virus has spread in the United States.

The virus is called HIV-2 (human immunodeficiency virus, type 2). That distinguishes it from the original AIDS virus, designated HIV-1.

Dr. Myron Essex, a researcher at Harvard University, has maintained the HIV-2 virus does not cause illness as severe or in the same frequency as the HIV-1 virus, a view disputed by researchers in the United States and France.

A screening test for HIV-2 has been developed and is awaiting approval by the U.S. Food and Drug Administration (FDA).

HIV-2, like HIV-1, is believed to be transmitted through sexual contact, blood transfusions, and contaminated hypodermic needles.

Also Wednesday, doctors urged that all patients at VD clinics should be tested for AIDS because a study showed a high incidence of infection in heterosexuals who did not believe they were at risk.

A study reported in the *New England Journal of Medicine*

AP, UPI News

Viruses

found patients at Baltimore's inner-city clinics for sexually transmitted diseases showed one-third of the men and nearly half of the women testing positive for the AIDS virus did not believe they were engaging in any high-risk behavior, researchers said.

The report said the rate of exposure to HIV-1 was 5.2 percent, or 209 of 4,028 clinic patients screened in Baltimore in early 1987.

AP and UPI News Services

AIDS Update: Third Virus Discovered

WASHINGTON — A third virus that causes AIDS has been found in Nigeria, Dr. Robert Gallo of the National Cancer Institute said Monday. But it may pose little or no threat outside Africa for now, Gallo said at the Third International Conference on AIDS, attended by 6,000 researchers from around the world.

Other research to be presented this week adds to evidence that the herpes virus can directly trigger the onset of AIDS in people infected with the AIDS virus.

"We now think a specific interaction may turn it on and leads to AIDS," Gallo said.

About 20 million people in the USA have been exposed to genital herpes. As much as 75 percent of the population — 180 million people — may have been exposed to two other herpes viruses — cytomegalovirus and Epstein-Barr — that also could act in concert with the AIDS virus. Both can be transmitted sexually and suppress the immune system.

Gallo, a top researcher, said of the new virus: "We don't know yet how wide it is spread or how actively it causes disease." It was found in 10 people who developed AIDS.

He also said a virus found years ago that causes a form of leukemia could — alone or in concert with the AIDS virus

Findlay, *USA Today* (June 2, 1987).

— cause the kind of immune suppression seen in AIDS patients.

He termed the phenomenon "double infection."

An unreleased Red Cross study of 30,000 blood donors has found that the leukemia-linked virus may be present in larger numbers of people than suspected. It may be even as widespread as the AIDS virus.

"If we confirm that it's as widespread as the AIDS virus, a new blood test could be necessary," said the Red Cross' Dr. Gerald Sandler.

Gallo said new studies show that despite the diversity of the viruses, they seem to have genetic similarities that would make one vaccine possible.

Stephen Findlay, *USA Today* (Copyright 1987, *USA Today*), June 2, 1987. Reprinted with permission.

A virus (such as HTLV-III) which successfully crosses the host-species barrier is often highly lethal to the new species (man in this case). A new virus which produces a persistent viraemia for life, and causes a slow virus encephalopathy (brain disease) after a mean incubation period of many years, would produce a lethal pandemic (very widespread infection) throughout the crowded cities and villages of the Third World of a magnitude unparalleled in human history. This is what the AIDS virus is now doing.

Dr. John Seale, former Consultant in Venereology at Middlesex and St. Thomas Hospitals, London, England. *Journal of the Royal Society of Medicine.*

Evidence of AIDS-related Virus Alarms Researchers

A potentially deadly AIDS-related virus is raising public health concerns in the United States after a preliminary survey found it showing up in donated blood at an alarming rate.

Detroit News (1987).

Viruses

The Food and Drug Administration has been urged to quickly help develop a simple, reliable test to screen blood for the virus HTLV-1.

The virus, structurally related to the acquired immune deficiency syndrome virus (HIV-1), is blamed for an epidemic of a deadly form of leukemia that surfaced in southern Japan in the late 1970s and an outbreak of paralyzing nerve disease in the Caribbean in the early 1980s.

It wasn't known that a virus was causing the illnesses until 1980 when Dr. Robert Gallo of the National Cancer Institute isolated HTLV-1.

The Centers for Disease Control in Atlanta and the National Cancer Institute in Washington said there is no known case of the new virus being transmitted in any blood donation in the United States.

But preliminary figures from an American Red Cross survey of six U.S. cities showed 10 carriers of the cancer-causing virus among 40,000 blood donors.

The cities involved in the survey were not disclosed for fear it would cause panic. However, sources revealed Atlanta was one of them and that none was in Michigan.

The type of leukemia blamed on the virus is called Adult T-cell leukemialymphoma. It is a blood and bone marrow cancer that kills within a year, with or without treatment.

The nerve disease, known as tropical spastic paraparesis, paralyzes and wastes the victim's legs and arms.

AIDS, which is fatal, attacks the body's immune system.

Dr. Jeanne Lusher, a Wayne State University professor and director of pediatric hematology at Children's Hospital, said incidence of HTLV-1 runs as high as 20 percent in blood samples taken in Jamaica and other parts of the Caribbean.

Sandler said public health officials are seeking a blood

Detroit News (1987).

screening test for HTLV-1 because of the lesson learned from AIDS.

"At a time when the virus is basically unknown to the United States, this is the time to develop a screening test for HTLV-1," he said.

Like the AIDS virus, HTLV-1 is passed by direct exposure to contaminated blood — through blood transfusion, shared hypodermic needles, sexual contact.

Sandler said the virus also is like AIDS in that infection is lifelong and the incubation period may be for decades.

The National Cancer Institute reports 74 known cases of Adult T-cell leukemialymphoma in this country, but there are no current figures on the number of deaths.

The incidence of tropical spastic paraparesis has been limited to the Caribbean area.

Dr. A. William Shafer, director of the Southeast Michigan Red Cross, said a rate of 10 cases of HTLV-1 carriers out of 40,000 donors, as reported from the blood bank meeting, would be alarming.

"If that's the case, it would be wise if we were to screen donors for this virus," Shafer said. "At the moment, there isn't such a test .... I'm concerned that the public will get hysterical."

Shafer said the FDA encouraged drug companies to develop a practical screening test for AIDS and he was confident such a test for HTLV-1 could be developed in six months to a year.

"This is another example of why the safest blood to receive is your own blood," Shafer said, referring to the practice of people storing their own blood for anticipated surgeries.

Susan Fleming, *The Detroit News*. Reprinted with permission of *The Detroit News*, a Gannett newspaper, copyright 1987.

Viruses

At the beginning of this treatise I mentioned that this would not be a religious presentation, but rather a secular study documented by international experts.

I believe I have accomplished my purpose; however, my calling by God would be a farce if I did not at least make a biblical statement in concluding my study.

Since I have quoted hundreds of specialists and reporters concerning temporal protection of life and body, let me now, as God's servant, present a few statements concerning the eternal welfare of one's soul. In doing so, let me repeat what I said as I ended my TV talk to all America and Canada on our TV special, "The AIDS Cover-Up."

God says, *Know ye not that the unrighteous shall not inherit the kingdom of God? Be not deceived: neither fornicators, nor idolators, nor adulterers, nor effeminate, nor abusers of themselves with mankind ... shall inherit the kingdom of God* (1 Corinthians 6:9,10).

The fornicators mentioned by God in this text are single folks who practice illicit sex outside of marriage during one-night stands or live-in relationships. Adulterers are married folks who do the same. The effeminate are young boys drawn into homosexual acts by the abusers of themselves with men — chicken hawks or life-long practicing homosexuals. Now, the God who does not practice discrimination says — all these groups who commit sexual sin outside of marriage, condom or no condom, are eternally excluded from eternal life unless they repent.

God again states, *Now the works of the flesh are manifest which are these; Adultery, fornication, uncleanness, lasciviousness* [the practice of sexual aberrations with greediness — never being satisfied ... THE RESULT: *They which do such things shall not inherit the kingdom of God* (Galatians 5:19,21).

On the basis of present statistics in this sex-crazed era, millions upon millions will be outside of God's Holy City forever because they flaunted, ignored, or ridiculed God's Holy Commandments. God said what He meant and meant what He said when, before the eyes of His servant Moses, He indelibly and eternally inscribed on a tablet of stone — *Thou shalt not commit adultery.*

Be like Moses. He decided to obey and follow God. He refused to enjoy the pleasures of sin for a season (see Hebrews 11:25). He made his decision centuries ago. Presently, he enjoys his eternal reward.

Some of us are like Moses, others are not. If not, is there hope for the fallen? Yes, beloved friend, and what I am about to say is exceedingly precious. Nothing I have said thus far can equal this next statement. Hear me. While AIDS blood contaminates others — the blood of Jesus Christ, God's Son, cleanses from all sin (see 1 John 1:7).

When our Saviour shed His precious efficacious blood upon Calvary's cross almost 20 centuries ago, that blood flowed to make the vilest offender of God's laws clean. I don't care what you have done, how often you have done it, how wicked, abominable, hideous, heinous, degraded, depraved, distorted, or defiled your sin was or is — hear me. The blood of Jesus Christ cleanseth from all sin. Praise the Lamb of God, which taketh away the sin of the world (see John 1:29). Hallelujah to Christ, who loved us and washed us from our sins in His own blood (see Revelation 1:5).

Can you be forgiven? Listen! *For God so loved the world, that he gave his only begotten Son, that whosoever* [whosoever — whosoever — you included] *believeth in him should not perish, but have everlasting life* (John 3:16). Will you come to Calvary today? Will you repent — change your mind about your lifestyle? Will you cast all your past and present sin upon Jesus? He longs to bear it.

Remember, Christ died for our sins — all of them. He wants to save you today, precious friend, if your heart is ready — if you want to be cleansed from the past — if you want your sins expiated, obliterated, and liquidated — if you want a new beginning, free from the hang-ups of the past, if you want to be saved, forgiven, cleansed, born again — then I want you to pray a special prayer with me. It doesn't take a lot to get saved. The thief on the cross prayed only nine words. Pray this prayer with me:

"Father, I'm a sinner. Thank You, Jesus, for shedding that precious, holy, sinless, untainted blood for me. I receive You now as my Saviour. Come into my heart. In Jesus' name. Amen."

Have you just asked Jesus to come into your heart? If you have, please write to us today. We would love to send you *First Steps in a New Direction* absolutely free. We want you to have help in those first new steps with Jesus Christ. So write to us and ask for *First Steps in a New Direction*.

Also, if you would like my book that provides a biblical analysis on AIDS, write and ask for *AIDS: 150 Million 1991*.

Other Books by Jack Van Impe

The Walking Bible
The "inside" story of Dr. Jack Van Impe. Forty years of the triumphs and tragedies of a remarkable man of God. New updated version includes new chapters and photographs. **$9**

Sin's Explosion
Though sin permeates and inundates the land, God specializes in bringing sinners to himself when sin is rampant. Includes scores of stirring quotes from great revival leaders. This book is a must for every library. **$9**

**Heart Disease in
Christ's Body**
Shocking! Explosive! Documented! A ringing defense of historic, biblical fundamentalism, proving that today's brand of fundamentalism differs from that of the founders, and a call for love and cooperation among all members of the body of Christ. **$7**

11:59 . . . and Counting!
What does the future hold for you and your loved ones? The questions that plague humanity are answered in this detailed account of mankind's march toward the Tribulation, Armageddon, and the hour of Christ's return. **$7**

Revelation Revealed
Re-released! Yes, you *can* understand what many consider to be the most complex book in the Bible. Dr. Van Impe's verse-by-verse teaching reveals the meaning of this prophetic treasure. **$7**

Israel's Final Holocaust
Over 240,000 in print! One of the most helpful explanations of Israel's role in end-time Bible prophecies ever published. What will the final holocaust be ... and how will it affect you? **$5**

ALCOHOL: The Beloved Enemy
Liquor and the Bible. Filled with wisdom and reasoning, this important book thoroughly covers the alcohol question. Includes historic background, current research, and statistics that may shock you. Bible help for a major problem. Every verse on the subject of wine from Genesis to Revelation is explained.

$5

Great Salvation Themes

Do you have unsaved loved ones . . . and don't know quite how to reach them? This book includes inspired messages by Dr. Van Impe that have been used to win thousands of souls through radio, TV, and citywide crusades. **$5**

The Baptism of the Holy Spirit

Dr. Van Impe's easy-to-understand study of who the Holy Spirit is, what He does, and why His baptism is for every believer. Includes what the Bible says about the personality, attributes, gifts, fruit, and power of the Holy Spirit. **$2**

God! I'm Suffering, Are You Listening?

Why do good people go through seemingly senseless suffering? Dr. Van Impe explains from a biblical perspective why even Christians suffer and the best way to make the most of misfortune. **$2**

The Happy Home: Child Rearing

Many parents are confused about how to raise their children to love and serve God. Dr. Van Impe provides sound Bible principles, as well as practical advice for raising children to be happy Christian adults. **$2**

America, Israel, Russia, and World War III

What will the end of the world be? Is a nuclear holocaust inevitable? Dr. Van Impe explains how Bible prophecy is being fulfilled, and the roles America, Israel, and Russia will play in the Battle of Armageddon. **$2**

Escape the Second Death

Five powerful salvation messages especially directed to the unsaved. A great witnessing tool. Explains the Bible way to be born again. (Excerpted from *Great Salvation Themes* .) **$2**

Exorcism and the Spirit World

What every Christian should know about Satan, demons, and demonic activity. Reveals the dangers of association with the occult, describes Satan worship, and tells how to defeat demon forces through the delivering power of the Holy Spirit. **$2**

The True Gospel

The only "good news" is that Christ died for our sins, was buried, and rose again. There is no other good news. Dr. Van Impe also covers Christ's last seven sayings upon the cross, and the importance of His resurrection. **$2**

Everything you always wanted to know about Prophecy

But didn't know who to ask! Dr. Van Impe answers questions on the Rapture, the Judgment seat of Christ, the Tribulation, and more. Headlines and international events interpreted in the light of Christ's soon return. This booklet will challenge you to live a life of holiness and service. **$2**

Can America Survive?

This dynamic book deals with where we've come from as a nation, where we are now, and what the future holds. Thoughtful, biblical answers for more than 30 compelling questions facing every concerned Christian today! **$2**

The Judgment Seat of Christ

Sheds light on the misunderstood subject of God's judgment. Covers the five judgments of the Bible, including the judgment of works, and a special section on the believer's crowns to be awarded on Judgment Day. **$2**

This Is Christianity

Millions who claim to be Christians — including church members — are not because they have never been born again. The message of this book will help you understand this vital subject and know what it means to be a follower of Christ. **$2**

The Cost of Discipleship and Revival

To be a true follower of Jesus Christ, the Bible says you must take up your cross and die to self. But just what kind of price do you have to pay? Find the answer, plus keys to revival, in the pages of this enlightening book. **$2**

What Must I Do To Be Lost?

Are you trusting in the traditions of men, your church, your good works? All the doctrines of the church will not get you into heaven. There is only one way to be saved — find out how in the pages of this book. **$2**

Religious Reprobates and Saved Sinners

A timely message by Dr. Van Impe that distinguishes "religion" from genuine salvation. If you've ever wondered how to separate the wolves from the sheep, you must read this frank, tell-it-like-it-is booklet! **$2**

AIDS: 150 Million 1991

Now in print! Contains the unedited transcript of the TV special, documenting the dangers of this deadly disease. A shocking exposé! **$2**

Order from: Jack Van Impe Ministries
Box J ● Royal Oak, Michigan 48068
In Canada: Box 1717, Postal Station A,
Windsor, Ontario N9A 6Y1

125407

JACK VAN IMPE MINISTRIES
ORDER FORM

QTY	DESCRIPTION	PRICE EACH	TOTAL
	AIDS IS FOR ~~LIFE~~ DEATH	$9	
	THE WALKING BIBLE	$9	
	SIN'S EXPLOSION	$9	
	HEART DISEASE IN CHRIST'S BODY	$7	
	11:59 . . . AND COUNTING!	$7	
	REVELATION REVEALED	$7	
	ISRAEL'S FINAL HOLOCAUST	$5	
	ALCOHOL: THE BELOVED ENEMY	$5	
	GREAT SALVATION THEMES	$5	
	THE BAPTISM OF THE HOLY SPIRIT	$2	
	GOD! I'M SUFFERING, ARE YOU LISTENING?	$2	
	THE HAPPY HOME: CHILD REARING	$2	
	AMERICA, ISRAEL, RUSSIA, AND WORLD WAR III	$2	
	ESCAPE THE SECOND DEATH	$2	
	EXORCISM AND THE SPIRIT WORLD	$2	
	THE TRUE GOSPEL	$2	

SUBTOTAL A

*ORDER FORM CONTINUED NEXT PAGE.

QTY	DESCRIPTION	PRICE EACH	TOTAL
	EVERYTHING YOU ALWAYS WANTED TO KNOW ABOUT PROPHECY	$2	
	THE JUDGMENT SEAT OF CHRIST	$2	
	THIS IS CHRISTIANITY	$2	
	THE COST OF DISCIPLESHIP AND REVIVAL	$2	
	WHAT MUST I DO TO BE LOST?	$2	
	RELIGIOUS REPROBATES AND SAVED SINNERS	$2	
	AIDS: 150 MILLION 1991	$2	

SUBTOTAL B

SUBTOTAL A

TOTAL AMOUNT ENCLOSED

NAME _____

ADDRESS _____

CITY _____ STATE _____ ZIP _____

Please tear out Order Form and send to:
  Jack Van Impe Ministries
  Box J • Royal Oak, Michigan 48068
  In Canada: Box 1717, Postal Station A
  Windsor, Ontario N9A 6Y1